Dear Reader,

The book you are holding came about in a rather different way to most others. It was funded directly by readers through a new website: Unbound. Unbound is the creation of three writers. We started the company because we believed there had to be a better deal for both writers and readers. On the Unbound website, authors share the ideas for the books they want to write directly with readers. If enough of you support the book by pledging for it in advance, we produce a beautifully bound special subscribers' edition and distribute a regular edition and ebook wherever books are sold, in shops and online.

This new way of publishing is actually a very old idea (Samuel Johnson funded his dictionary this way). We're just using the internet to build each writer a network of patrons. At the back of this book, you'll find the names of all the people who made it happen.

Publishing in this way means readers are no longer just passive consumers of the books they buy, and authors are free to write the books they really want. They get a much fairer return too – half the profits their books generate, rather than a tiny percentage of the cover price.

If you're not yet a subscriber, we hope that you'll want to join our publishing revolution and have your name listed in one of our books in the future. To get you started, here is a £5 discount on your first pledge. Just visit unbound.com, make your pledge and type **elephant5** in the promo code box when you check out.

Thank you for your support,

Dan, Justin and John
Founders, Unbound

DEATH AND THE ELEPHANT

DEATH AND THE ELEPHANT

RAZ SHAW

How Cancer Saved My Life

Unbound

This edition first published in 2018

Unbound
6th Floor Mutual House, 70 Conduit Street, London W1S 2GF
www.unbound.com

Raz Shaw, 2018

Music notes p.20 reproduced from 'Amazing Grace'

Tally marks image pp.76–77 © Marie Maerz, Shutterstock.com

Text Design by PDQ

A CIP record for this book is available from the British Library

ISBN 978-1-78352-477-8 (trade hbk)
ISBN 978-1-78352-478-5 (ebook)
ISBN 978-1-78352-476-1 (limited edition)

Printed in Great Britain by Clays Ltd, St Ives Plc

1 3 5 7 9 8 6 4 2

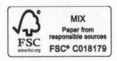

MIX
Paper from
responsible sources
FSC® C018179

This book is dedicated in part to the amazing Royal Marsden Hospital and so, vicariously, to the NHS. On 5 July 1950, Aneurin Bevan launched the National Health Service on three core principles:

1. That it meets the needs of everyone.
2. That it be free at the point of delivery.
3. That it be based on clinical need, not ability to pay.

It's a remarkable testimony to this country that, despite repeated attempts to undermine those core principles, they held strong in 1995 and they still, to some degree, do so to this day.

That's not politics, or trumpet-blowing, that's just something that we take for granted and need to remind ourselves of now and again. Before I was diagnosed in 1995, I certainly hadn't really given it much thought.

To Val Shaw aka my mum

For her unwavering, unconditional, unequivocal and too often underappreciated support.

With special thanks to the Patrons who supported this book

Anna Aleff
Michael Alexander
Bill & Siân Buckhurst
Claire Cooper
Amber Evans
Phoebe Fox
Terence Frisch
Marguerite Galizia
Harry Hepple
Julie Hesmondhalgh
Sam Heughan
Anthony Horowitz
Polly Hubbard
Janey Johnson
Jack Knowles
Richard Lee
Julie Legrand
Bruce McLeod
Andrea Neumann-Claus
Debbie Oates
Kate Plantin
Charlie Russell
Gesine Schmücker-Schüßler
Mark Shaw
Henry Shields
Rich and Nia Smith
Naomi Wallace
Lucinda Westcar
Chris White

CONTENTS

THOSE WHO DIDN'T MAKE IT

I wanted to write this book in honour of those who didn't make it. One in three of us gets cancer. I don't know what the survival rates are. All I know is that nothing makes me sadder than when someone dies from this evil disease. I didn't feel as strongly as that before I entered the club. The cancer club. Those deaths didn't seem so personal. But I joined the club – and it *is* a club – and in this club we should feel impacted every time we hear of someone not making it. And whether they lived through cancer for a day, a week, a year, ten years or a lifetime before they died, this book is an attempt to glory in those moments of living. I am not down with the phrase 'cancer survivor'. It makes me feel a bit sick in my mouth. Not completely sure why. It is something to do with it unwittingly disrespecting those who didn't survive. As if those people had failed in some fashion. Yet *they*, to me, are the brave ones. The rest of us are just people who are still living, for now. Not only do they not have the luxury of living, but the pain of their death goes on in the loved ones they leave behind. That's the part that makes me saddest. And that to me has been the most important thing to remember when writing this book. I can make light of my own life and my cancer journey. Because it's just that. *My* life. But I can't make light of yours and I can't make light of those who didn't have the luxury of surviving. I hope they would have appreciated, understood and enjoyed this book.

PREFACE

I was twenty-eight years old when I was diagnosed with cancer. I am now fifty.

Spoiler Alert: I don't die in the end. At least not in the first edition.

This isn't a book about how to survive cancer. That would just be weird. And wrong.

This is a book about having cancer and a gambling addiction both at the same time. And coping and not coping and trying to cope. It's not about tomorrow. It is solely about today. Trying to cope today. What happens tomorrow is for tomorrow.

If I had the opportunity to go back in time, I wouldn't change a thing.

Despite the hideousness of chemo. Despite the endless days of exhausted inertia. Despite having a head the size of a pumpkin and a neck the size of Hulk Hogan's thigh. Despite it taking me out of the loop of the world and making me feel a boy again. Despite the hidden loneliness. Despite being almost eaten alive by the monster that is addiction. Despite the constant soft rumble of low-level despair.

Despite. Despite. Despite. Despite. Despite. Despite. Despite.

It's somewhat of a cliché to say that the journey through cancer treatment and gambling addiction and out the other side has made me who I am today. But it happens to be true. It has given me jewels of insight and afforded me the privilege of sometimes being someone else's shoulder to lean or cry on. And the writing of this book has thrown up questions that

I had never before thought to ask myself. The biggest and most obvious being: has that simultaneous journey through and beyond cancer and gambling addiction changed me? My outlook and personality? And the answer has to be yes. Without a doubt. I have no placebo 'me' to compare me to, so I have no true ability to gauge in what way and by how much. And that's a big reason why I wanted to write this book. To find out. It's a big reason why I wanted my twenty-eight-year-old self and my fifty-year-old self to communicate in some fashion. To find out.

The other almost impossible question to answer is how present has cancer been in my life these last twenty-two years, and how involved is it still in everything I do, say or think? That *is* an impossible question, but what I do know is that it's present enough for me to want to write a book about it. It's present enough for me to want to share some personal insights into what it felt like living with it. And it's present enough to have given me an awareness and an insight into life and death that I would never have properly gleaned without it. And that's the gift that keeps on giving.

It's also important to say that this is a book that doesn't demand that you be strong. Or that you weep oceans. When I was ill there were times I was happy to talk about it and times I wasn't. There were moments when I was open and honest, and lots of moments when it was easier to bury my head in the sand. The cancer sand. It wasn't always a breeze. It was often a hurricane. But being in the eye of a hurricane can be fun sometimes even if at the same time it's somewhat life-threatening.

Part of living is the thrill of confronting death and saying: '*Do your worst, motherfucker.*'

Sometimes death wins and sometimes it doesn't, but always, *always*, it is better to have stood up to it and tried to find moments of joy within it than to have simply held up your hands and given in to it.

And you never stop absorbing stuff and learning stuff. And real life never ceases to surprise you. Every day.

Just before my self-imposed rewriting deadline, something happened that forced me away from my self-reflection for a nanosecond to think about someone else. Someone else! Goddammit. Worse still, that someone else wasn't just any someone else, it was THE someone else. Or should I say SHE someone else.

Everybody needs an unconditional when they are ill. Unconditionals put up with your shit. Sometimes literally. Unconditionals keep the unwanteds at bay. Unconditionals step forward or back without you having to ask. Unconditionals treat you to food that has proper taste at posh Harvey Nichols-type places to take away the psychological pain of a syringe. Unconditionals come in many forms. Mine came in three letters.

MUM.

I am the youngest of three boys. That has afforded me a rollercoaster of favouritism and neglect. I always thought the hardest thing about being a parent must be NOT having favourites, but as I got older I realised that OF COURSE parents have favourites. How could they not? The secret about good parenting is not SHOWING that favouritism to those self-same kids.

I happened to have two parents in two different schools of thought on that. I had a father who had no ability or even desire to hide his feelings about his children, and, as luck wouldn't have it, I happened to *not* be top of the tots. In fact, out of his three sons, I'm not sure I even made the top three.

This isn't the right arena to go into deep analysis about the reasons why, and it's certainly not my intention to disparage him. Publicly, at least. In fact, just the opposite. Since his death a few years ago I have managed to find some rationale for what at the time seemed unfair and upsetting.

It's about **relatability**. The older I got, and the more I started to discover who I was, the less my father could relate to me. A young Jewish north London boy should be interested in... I don't know what? Not arty things anyway. I should have read the signs when twelve-year-old me was leading the choir in the school carol service. I strode proudly and purposefully down the aisle of the church, in my cassock and ruff, and belted out the first verse of 'Once in Royal David's City'. My Jewish father shifted uncomfortably on his wooden pew, not knowing whether to be proud or ashamed. It seems to me that contradiction stayed with him, about me, for the rest of his life and he had no filter with which to hide it. In simple terms, I have grown to accept that my father loved me but didn't like me. Such is life.

My mother, on the other hand, has always sailed the seas of fairness brilliantly. She had/has three very different sons and that in itself surely presents a challenge. It's only natural that the personality of one of those three would appeal more to a person than the other two. Hard to resist my winning spoilt brat youngest child charm, of course, but it wouldn't necessarily have to be me! Well, one way or the other, I can honestly say that my mother has never revealed her favouritism cards. Or at least, if she has, I was never able to detect them. And that's a huge skill. Having said that, these days all three of us have been relegated. She has one favourite son. And his name is Andy Murray. Or Sir Andy as he's now known. The boy can do no wrong. I mean. Andy, c'mon, you have your own mum. And she's pretty hot is Judy. Leave mine alone!

And that leads me to the point.

The mother. *My* mother.

Just before settling down to write the final draft of this book, my mother was diagnosed with lung cancer. Pretty much out of the blue. It was naturally quite a shock and it provoked within me surprising emotions. Considering the essence of this book is about emotional contradictions when dealing with a cancer diagnosis, this news took any wind I might have had out of my balding sails. Everything I have written and talked about as far as my illness is concerned has been connected with trying to break down the taboos of the C word. Or CA, as hospitals seem to call it these days, presumably to soften the cancer word. And that's CA as in the separate letters C.A. (C&A without the 'and' or the eighties fashions), as opposed to CA as in car. I think the idea being that breaking it down to just the letters makes it somewhat impersonal and thus more palatable. Hmm. Not sure I agree. Anyway, the point is that dealing with my own CA was much easier than hearing about my mother's. All the things I preach on a daily basis, 'cancer doesn't equal death' etc., flew out of the window, and I found myself in deep reflection on life and what it would be like to lose my mother. I was more than surprised at how profoundly it had affected me. I don't know why I was surprised. This was my mother, for fuck's sake. I think maybe I had thought that dealing with my own illness and gambling addiction and coming out the other side and then preaching to others about it had given me some kind of superpower. The Grim-Sweeper-Man (he can sniff out and sweep up an emotional tragedy in the blink of his super-heroic eye). But my mother's illness showed me that that clearly isn't true and that I have an infinite way to go before I graduate to superhero status.

What *is* true is that back in the day my life had been going nowhere. I was a gambling addict desperately searching for help. For direction. For a purpose and focus.

On 13 June 1995, the day after my twenty-eighth birthday, I found it.

That day, I was diagnosed with non-Hodgkin's lymphoma.

Or to be medically accurate: **stage 4 sclerosing mediastinal non-Hodgkin's lymphoma of the large cell type.**

AKA: cancer of the lymph glands.

And cancer saved my life.

PROLOGUE

When I started writing this book, I tried to chart a potted version of my life history up to the point of the 1995 diagnosis so as to give you some idea of who you're dealing with here, but every time I tried to write it, it just felt too literal and linear. And as a theatre director, literal and linear are dirty, dirty words. They are one-star words.

So instead I have been searching for the connection between the four-year-old me, the eleven-year-old me, the teenage me and the twenty-something me. Apart from the fact that they were all me, of course. And then I remembered something that happened in the last rehearsal room I was in. Well, less what happened but more what someone said. To me.

I was directing a play called *WIT* at the Royal Exchange Theatre in Manchester. It is no accident that *WIT* uses cancer as its central means to explore human behaviour in the face of adversity. I had wanted to direct that play for about as long as I have been thinking about writing this book. The lead character, a professor of metaphysical poetry dying of ovarian cancer, was played by the sublime (sublime actor and even more sublime human being) Julie Hesmondhalgh. We didn't really know each other before we started rehearsals. Casting is always a crapshoot. Not just in terms of whether that actor is right for that part but, just as importantly, whether you might bring the best out of each other or not.

Turns out Julie and I had great rehearsal-room chemistry. That doesn't necessarily mean that we always got along but that's all part of it. The dialectic materialism of theatre (I did politics A level. Am showing off. I only got a C, though, so…).

In layman's terms, as long as you ultimately respect each other and believe in each other, then a clash of opinions can often lead to THE answer. An answer that you may never have come up with without such a clash. Julie and I revelled in these clashes. It was our creative spark.

One day, I can't remember the context, but I must have been pushing Julie quite hard (Julie's bravery knows no bounds) as she suddenly turned to me and in her deep Accrington burr said:

'I can't go there. I am not like you. You love feeling uncomfortable. You fucking revel in it.'

Wow!

OK!

We had only known each other a couple of weeks and she had already spotted my tell. A tell I didn't really know I had until it was pointed out to me at that moment. And she was right. I DO revel in it.

In what?

I think I revel in challenging myself to see if I can deal with a situation I have never dealt with before. Or, put more literally, I don't really feel alive if I am not slightly churning up inside. More than that, without it I am often just plain bored. That churning is the springboard to my urgency and activity, and it's the thing that keeps me alert and interested. In other words, it's my fuel. My adrenaline. Anyone who knows me will say, 'No shit, Sherlock. That's the least shocking discovery since finding out that Barry Manilow was gay.'

But to me it was a bit of a revelation. Yes, I knew adrenaline was a long-term companion of mine but I never realised how close we'd been from a very early age. That discovery also explains how I ended up normalising it. I needed that churning-up-inside sensation to feel normal and even-keeled. So it became my petrol AND my tranquiliser all at the same time. A contradiction with which a therapist would have a field day.

THE FIRST SNIFF OF ADRENALINE

It was 1971. I was four years old. I was called Darren back then; that was the name my folks misguidedly chose to give me. I was the youngest of three boys. The son of Val and Norman Shaw. Val had a lingerie boutique called Chica. I am not saying that spending my early childhood rummaging through Playtex Cross Your Heart bras and high-waisted lacy panty briefs affected me at all, but I am not saying it didn't either. Norman was an East End tailor and fledgling property tycoon. We holidayed where most up and coming north London Jews holidayed. Torremolinos, of course! Where else!

In the Torremolinos hotel we had interconnecting rooms to the parents. I had the put-you-up bed. I always had the put-you-up bed. And the hand-me-down clothes. There are many perks to being the youngest of three, but at four years old I had yet to find them. It made me different, though, and I am certain that if I could remember what I thought back then, a bit of me quite liked that.

Anyway, to cut a long story quite short. A hotel fell on us. A Torremolinos hotel to be precise! It *was* quite an event. An event that could warrant almost a whole chapter, but, in the spirit of brevity, here are the highlights. In useful and easy-to-read bullet points.

- North London family stay at four-star hotel in Torremolinos.
- Three boys aged four, seven and nine go down to breakfast alone, leaving their parents to do whatever parents do when left alone in a hotel room without their annoying kids.
- The three boys have their breakfast and then go and sit on a sofa in the lounge-type area.
- The ceiling to the lounge-type area collapses due to bulldozers on the roof being used to construct a tennis court.
- The sofa, with all three boys on it, falls two floors.

- Val and Norman finish whatever they are doing and head down for breakfast.
- Val and Norman take the stairs as the lift is out of order.
- On arriving at the ground floor, Val and Norman find devastation in the annexe area equivalent to the disaster movie *Earthquake*. Although that film isn't out till 1974 so it's not a reference that would have occurred to them. Not that they would necessarily be searching for movie parallels at that particular moment.
- Eight hours and three dead bodies later (this IS a real-life disaster movie), there is still no sign of the three boys.
- Val and Norman fear the worst.
- In desperation, Norman points out to the rescue workers (tabloid term) a place where the three boys used to sit on a sofa watching a painter paint.
- The rescue workers dig there and lower themselves down twenty feet.
- They shout. The boys shout back. The sofa has landed in an air pocket formed by a felled pillar, thus saving the three boys' lives.
- The rescue workers rescue the boys. Hence the term 'rescue workers'.
- The last to be carried out of the rubble-filled air pocket is four-year-old Darren Shaw. He is wearing natty swimming trunks. He has pissed all over them. He is four. Give him a break!
- The crowd cheers as he is led into the ambulance.

And the crowd did cheer. And I think I remember not being totally averse to the cheering. And I do remember thinking that the whole thing was more exciting than scary. And that was my first taste of adrenaline. Apart from the underwear rummaging, of course. And my first taste of defaulting into almost flat-lining when everyone else was a bit overwhelmed.

Being somewhat underwhelmed in the midst of much drama is a curiously calm and empowering place to be. It was the first glimpse of a strange phenomenon that I am only now beginning to identify. Namely, searching for a place of high adrenaline IN ORDER to do everything I can to undermine it and undercut it. No, it doesn't really make sense to me either. It's like the weird beauty of swimming underwater. The big world banging on up there, but me in peace and in otherworldly calmness down here. Until the need for breath has to rear its ugly head and spoil everything!

And for a few days after that, we were fifteen-minute celebrities. All over the tabloids. We were called the Chicos de Dios. Children of God.

Well.

Yes.

Possibly.

And all the playing up to the press cameras and stuff just seemed like loads of fun to this peculiar child. And it turns out that being the youngest DOES have some perks. I was the one chosen for all the '*back in the arms of his mother*' shots! Result. Speak to my agent!

I have no idea whether that was the seed and the spark that led to me being a gambling addict, and/or it was the germ of a personality that oddly enjoyed the trials of dealing with stage 4 cancer; but the connection is definitely there, and reconnecting with that four-year-old brat is certainly eye-opening.

ADRENALINE AT ELEVEN

I was eleven years old.

Pee-pants-hotel-falling-on-top-of-me trauma was well behind me.

At eleven years old I made a horrific discovery. A discovery that would skew the next twenty years of my life. I loved gambling. I mean, I discovered gambling and loved it. As opposed to waking up one day and thinking, 'You know what, I love gambling.'

In 1978 my parents took my brothers and me for supper at the Wimbledon dog track. We sat and had our meal next to a window looking directly onto the track. We ate our food and the waiter would come round and take our drinks order and at the same time take our bets for that particular race. I didn't know it then but this was posh gambling. It was never like this again!

I'll have a glass of cream soda and two whole pounds on trap five, please, waiter.

Posh!

I wasn't legally allowed to bet. I was eleven. But I did. Bet.

And I won.

I WON!!

I won fifteen pounds.

Fifteen whole pounds.

FIFTEEN!

Yes! Yes! Yes! Yes! Yes! Yes! Yes! Yes! Yes! Yes! Yes! Yes! Yes! Yes! Yes!

I remember it vividly. An adrenaline buzz that felt unlike anything I had experienced before. An eleven-year-old with adrenaline gushing out of every pore and pimple.

A year later I was taken to Vegas. Viva, Viva Las Vegas! With last year's trackside rush still firmly lodged in my memory Vegas was adrenaline heaven. And it swirled around me like it was designed to. This was old-school Vegas. Late seventies Vegas. *Goodfellas* Vegas. Big suits and glitter. Big hair and Joe Pesci. And that was just my family.

And moving walkways. And no sunlight. And an amazing soundscape.

And to a twelve-year-old who was unwittingly searching for somewhere to belong, this was it. Stark lighting, buzzers, bells and seedy sex.

It was all so wonderfully awful. So wonderfully other worldly. Awful and wonderful and weird. And so so right. Daylight was the enemy. I was twelve but I instinctively knew that every second NOT spent in the casino was a second wasted. And I wasn't gambling. I was too young. But I was taking it all in:

- The slightly rancid and musty twenty-four-hour tang in the air.
- The sterile laughter-free zone.
- The random yelps of the craps dealers.
- The multi-toned beeps of the fruit machines.
- The zero-skirted over-made-up cocktail waitresses.
- The free stale sandwiches.

If I knew then how much that kernel of a feeling would grow into something beyond my control, I may have been able to cut it off at its source. But I didn't. I just felt it. And it was horribly thrilling.

In the evenings my father and my oldest brother would go and see an adult show. Whatever that was. My mother and I would stay behind in the hotel. The Caesar's Palace Hotel. Complete with those space-age walkways and banks of mirrors. Filled with the sound of men and women nervously shuffling their gambling chips, croupiers shouting gobbledegook and bells seeming to go off all round you followed by dull almost apologetic cheers. This was more than my twelve-year-old future addict's heart could possibly desire.

My mum was a little bit of a gambler. That's where I got it from. She always did have something of a predilection for a casino. And for a fruit machine in particular. Fruit machines are hypnotic. They are designed that way. Hypnosis combined with sporadic bursts of adrenaline. That way addiction lies. Some thirty years later I devised and directed a play about the adrenaline of that addiction. (See Appendix 2.) If only twelve-year-old me had been taking notes. Instead he yearned to pull the lever and press the flashing buttons.

My mum loved pulling and pressing. So to speak. Every time she did, the woman, my mother, became a girl, my mother. It was a fantastic equaliser between us. I stood with her for ages, and now and then – when the casino people weren't looking – she let me lean into the machine and pull that magical lever. My insides lit up much like the machines themselves. Time disappeared and, in that moment, a huge part of my life was mapped out. And it's nobody's fault. Not my mother's, not society's, not mine. (Well, more mine than any of the other lot, but not completely mine!) Something triggered inside me that remained resident for almost twenty years.

TEENAGE ADRENALINE KICKS

It was around that time that I discovered that I saw life in a slightly less regular way than the next child. The last few years of my prep school were amazing. I was eleven/twelve/thirteen. I had discovered this personality that could be cheeky rather than naughty, that could interact with people much older than me and that could make people laugh. The low point of those years was, of course, not being cast as Queen Elizabeth I in the school play. A classic casting error. I could have brought so many more dimensions to that woman than Mark Dingemans did! Where the fuck is he now? I was truly bruised by that (that's not hyperbole, I am ashamed to say that I actually was). I vowed to show them that they were wrong.

MR BATES, PART ONE

The high point of that time was my friendship/adoration/ slight non-sexual obsession with my English/PE teacher Mr Bates (leave it). When I look back at it now, he was the first adult to truly treat me as an individual. He was the first adult who really listened to me and who seemed to care about what came out of my mouth. He was the first adult who made me feel unique. He made me feel like a young man who didn't warrant being talked down to or patronised or undermined. I am not saying I was a special boy. Just the opposite. His genius as a teacher was that he had identified something that, for whatever reason, was lacking in me, and he made it his mission to try to find different ways to fuel that half-empty childish soul. He would talk to me at length about life and about philosophical things. He would allow me licence to express myself in a way nobody had ever done before and not many have since.

It used to upset me and anger me that other pupils and some teachers used to find our friendship a bit suspect. His 'guardianship' was totally unconditional, completely devoid of any subtext and absolutely on the level. He was the first person who recognised that I might be seeing life from a slightly different angle to others. He continually encouraged me to express rather than suppress that side of my personality. The unconventional side. That was huge for me. To this day I don't think I have ever been as creative or articulate as at that time. And it was all down to that one person teaching me the power of saying yes rather than no.

And that has lived with me ever since. It played a huge part in my cancer journey. It helped me accept things even though they were often incredibly difficult, demanding and depressing. It helped me see today as the point. Not yesterday or tomorrow.

TODAY

I realise now that everything Mr Bates was trying to teach me was about trying to accept who you are **today**. What you have to offer **today**. What you want **today**. Accept it, confront it and say yes to it. He did it just by talking to me and seeming to take me seriously. This acceptance from an adult that I idolised felt good. And for a brief moment I think I experienced happy. I think? Yes.

THE POWER OF THE YES

Yes is something I too easily forget to put into practice in my now life, sometimes only remembering its power when it's too late.

It was something that I absolutely instinctively armed myself with when I was diagnosed. The power of the Yes was a simple gateway to the slightly less tangible concept of positivity. I guess that's why I am covering my early years in this book. Those were days when my window to all the grace in the world was still fairly wide open, and so anything I was given then has pretty much stayed with me till now.

And Yes is a powerful tool to be given.

Yes? **Yes? Yes!**

MR BATES, PART TWO

Mr Bates was both an English teacher and a sports teacher so he ticked both my boxes of interest. He was also a little bit naughty. Which I liked. I have always been attracted to naughty people. He was having a 'scandalous' affair with the mother of one of my friends. I loved him even more for that. He had a Kevin Keegan perm. I loved him so much for that, that I got a perm to match. On top of my Jew-fro! At the age of twelve!

And to top it all, on a school skiing trip to Italy he managed to schmooze the hotel chef into letting us into his kitchen to watch Arsenal v Valencia in the European Cup Winners' Cup Final on the only telly in the hotel (this was 1980). We lost on penalties. My other hero of that time, Liam Brady, missed a penalty. Losing was disappointing but I was so overcome by the exhilaration and adrenaline of the whole exceptional event that I hardly noticed the result. In fact, I remember skipping to the disco where my classmates had been while Mr Bates and I were watching the match. Me? Skipping? Those *must* have been happy days. And that euphoria must have translated into twelve-year-old sex appeal because just two hours later I was having my first kiss at the bottom of the hotel steps with a girl older and taller than me! This was adrenaline plus! Could life get any better than this?

Well, no actually. Those remain the happiest two years of my life.

HOME IS WHERE THE ART IS

And it was indeed all downhill from there.

The first time I felt my soul die a little was at the age of thirteen when I was sitting my mock Common Entrance exams. Common Entrance, to those who don't know, is the gateway from posh junior school to posh senior school. I think the first exam I took was geography. For me geography was an extremely dreary middling subject. I could do English. Or at least I had an interest in it. I had zero interest in the sciences. None. Not even biology! Geography seemed to me to be the love child of English and science. I should have been able to get at least somewhere with it. It was when I read the first question that it hit me. Right in the gut. It wasn't that the question didn't make sense or even that I couldn't have had some reasonable stab at it; it was just that it was the first time I realised that I wasn't equipped with enough academic clarity to get to the heart of that question.

CLARITY

Clarity is absolutely the key to academic intelligence. Without that clarity I didn't have the tools or the insight to scribe a reasoned and articulate argument that would ultimately warrant top marks. At that moment I realised that it takes both measured clarity and a methodical but sponge-like brain to be conventionally intelligent. At that moment I realised that that could never and would never be me. At that moment I discovered **sad** for the first time. Sad because I knew this exam and the rest of my school life were going to be a bigger academic struggle than I ever thought they would be. And deeper sad as I knew that I was never going to 'sparkle' with intellectual notoriety. A notoriety that I had secretly craved.

And that sadness, buried deep in my soul, has been my constant companion ever since. That sadness has been my creative driving force, too. It has forced me to be always searching for something that I can do as well, if not better, than others. Something that I can completely own. Something I can hold on to that might make me feel uniquely me. And, one chilly April afternoon in 1982, I found it.

I was fifteen. A boy in chaos. Trying and failing to find his own identity. His USP, if you like. Being threatened with an enforced school move as it was evident he was in full drift mode. Of course it didn't help that I had two brothers with big personalities who preceded me at the same school. It was the first time I found that I didn't like being compared to anyone else. Still don't. I was just another of the Shaws. '*Oh no, not another bloody Shaw*' was the recurring schoolmaster refrain. So

I fought and fought and fought against it. I wasn't aware that I was fighting. I just knew I didn't fit. Anywhere.

Then the epiphany happened.

I walked into Dyne House auditorium. The school theatre. I sat on the back row and watched a rehearsal taking place. It wasn't immediate. It wasn't a metaphorical bolt of lightning. It was just a slow melding into belonging. I can't remember what the rehearsal was or even why I was there but I can remember the odd but beautiful feeling of discovery that I had found my club. My world. And to this day, every time I find myself in a darkened, almost empty theatre, normally about to start a tech, I catch myself and recollect that feeling and am reminded of the lost fifteen-year-old uncovering his very own Neverland. A place where being different was an asset not an oddity. And uniqueness was encouraged as it was at the heart of creativity.

At the centre of my new life-changing world was English teacher and theatre director Philip Swan. He was one of those brilliant teachers who loved what he did, loved discovering the individual in the boy and loved coaxing and sometimes bullying the talent out of you. He helped me bring out the *me* in me again. He introduced me to a world that made sense and a world that I knew I would call home for the rest of my life. And within that environment I thrived. Not academically. That was always a bit of a chore. But I thrived as a person and the man that I instinctively knew I eventually wanted to be began to emerge.

I say 'began' because it took a hiatus of fourteen years, a university course I despised, some jobs that made me feel more than ill, a raging gambling addiction and a cancer journey, before the man in me started to find his feet in the real world.

It is, oddly, both a blessing and a curse to discover at the age of fifteen what you should be doing for the rest of your life. While it takes the lid off the pressure of the search, at the same time it means that when you are NOT doing that thing, the pain is immediate and profound and lasts for as long as you are not doing it.

And that pain did run deep. Sometimes still does.

At sixteen, I was even more sure that I had discovered what I had been put on this earth to do. Problem was that I was doubly certain that the paternal battle against me doing it would be full on and seemingly never ending. I wish now that I had had more of a stomach for that particular fight. When you are *sure* that academia and university are not your thing **and** yet you find yourself at university and not drama school, you just know it's not going to end well.

But at the time it seemed easier and less emotionally painful than the alternative. The alternative being having to listen to one irrational and insensitive reason after another from my father as to why I should ignore my heart and listen to his head. The twisted, knotted-up agony of not being listened to by him was too much for me to deal with back then. Much easier to convince myself that going to university *would* be a good idea and wouldn't be a TOTAL waste of my time!

So studying Business Organisation at Heriot-Watt University in Edinburgh rather than being at drama school in London was where I could be found in the winter of 1986. Miles away – geographically, emotionally and literally – from what I knew I should be doing.

The displacement that I felt meant I was looking for something to fill that void inside me. Subconsciously, you understand. If I had been in a fully functioning conscious state, I would have been on the first overnight sleeper back to London. I don't think I properly woke up till the diagnosis some ten years later.

I found that something in the strange world of blue-rinse-populated Lothian Road amusement arcades by day and seedy Edinburgh casinos by night. It was the perfect escape. And at midnight every night – for its army of Chinese customers – the casino laid on a full and free Chinese buffet. That was my justification. It was free. I was a student. And a Jew! It was free. Free. Food. Free food! I couldn't turn that down. I would even invite my friends along to experience the gratis gourmet Chinese experience. However, gambling is a solitary pastime. At least gambling addiction is. So I would encourage my friends to leave soon after they had filled themselves up on the perfumed grease. I, on the other hand, would stay. For hours. Now and again I would win. Sometimes I would win big. Most of the time I would lose. A lot of the time I would lose big. Most nights I would leave the casino at 4 a.m. realising that the free Chinese buffet I had had four hours earlier was the most expensive Chinese meal of my life.

Being a gambling addict on a student grant was not sustainable so I had to become really well versed in the art of lying to the parents to justify why I needed them to give me any more money. I was an expert at it. Addiction and lying go together like peaches and cream.

When I left university, I made a desperate effort to be the person I knew I was meant to be, so I went to drama school and took a one-year postgraduate diploma in acting. My gambling took a back seat. For the first year or so out of drama school I was actually almost happy. I was acting a bit and that was satiating me to some degree. But as the acting dried up so did the money, and I turned to my old friend gambling for company. It would win me my fortune, you see, and that fortune would enable me to take even more control over my life and become a theatre director. The job I secretly craved. But the odd thing is that you need money to gamble, so I had to ditch the dream and find a job that paid big.

A few years earlier in a surreal university holiday job, I discovered I had the unenviable gift of being able to sell stuff. Timeshare in Menorca to be precise. I know! As if my soul hadn't been sullied enough already. So now, in order to fuel my addiction, I reminded myself of that 'talent' and took a part-time job selling light bulbs and industrial cleaning chemicals over the telephone. It was a slippery slope and I slid down it effortlessly. The addiction devil on my shoulder urging me to descend. Three years later my creativity had been completely swallowed up, my soul had long been extinguished, and I found myself earning a small fortune running a dodgy telesales company in London. That small fortune never stayed a fortune for very long. My gambling was out of control. My wallet was always empty. For the last year of that job my chest ached every morning as I sat on the Tube going to work. An ache so deep that a number of times I literally couldn't breathe. I was festering in my own casino sweat of addiction, and escape was a luxury I didn't deserve. And then real life put its gnarly hand on my shoulder.

PART ONE:
THE DIAGNOSIS

12 JUNE 1995

It was Monday, 12 June 1995. My twenty-eighth birthday. I was a lost, directionless gambling addict.

Three weeks earlier I had quit my highly paid telesales job. My friend Debbie had written a play. She knew that I was trapped in the vicious circle of highly paid job/gambling addiction. So she asked me to direct it. Her play that is. On one condition. That I devoted *all* my time to it. Full-time, in other words.

The moment she said it, I could feel the relief course through my bones. I said yes. And yes. And yes. I phoned up and resigned from my job that instant. A phone call that changed my life. I stepped into that petrifying void of the unknown. The pain in my chest vanished immediately.

However, three weeks later a new pain appeared. This was no '*I hate my life*' pain. This was a real pain. An actual physical pain.

PINEAPPLE HEAD

It had all happened so quickly. One bright summer morning, I woke up with a neck the size of a pineapple on steroids. It wasn't a good look. To make matters worse, when I bent down all the blood rushed to my neck (for once!) and I found it impossible to breathe. Which is always tricky. My head wanted to explode, and my skin felt like it was searching for a way to break away from my body and release the mini blood tsunami brewing up inside me.

For a few days I kidded myself that my inability to breathe and my huge throbbing neck might be the result of an allergic reaction to something I'd eaten. It was much easier to kid myself than to face up to the truth. The truth that there might be something seriously wrong with me. So I spent three long breathless days in glorious avoidance mode. I don't like doctors at the best of times. I think it's an authority thing. And an 'out of control' thing. Plus, it took me back to school medicals when the elderly male doctor would cup my balls and ask me to cough. I was never sure when to cough. Just before he cupped my balls? Just after? And I certainly wasn't sure *why* he cupped my balls at all!

After three days of medical evasion, it seemed clear to me that unless I had eaten a whole pineapple which had then lodged itself in my neck, there probably was something really wrong with me.

THAT VOICE

Eventually, I dragged myself off to my GP. He drew some diagrams that I didn't understand and sent me for an X-ray **THAT INSTANT**. When I felt that cold X-ray plate against my chest, I got a strange piercing premonition of what was to come. I chose to ignore it.

The next day I returned to the doctor, who was in receipt of the results.

I knew something was up when he put that voice on. You know that voice. The one that comes through a faint smile and sounds like a cross between a Radio 4 continuity announcer and someone giving their best phone sex chat (not that I'd know what that sounds like).

A breathy gravitas.

'There's a shadow between your lungs. I think you should go and have a biopsy **TOMORROW***.'*

That *'tomorrow'* was not soft and breathy. It was sharp and shouty and made me jump. It was a subtly unsubtle way of saying:

4

'CANCER, I THINK IT'S CANCER.'

So I toddled off to have my chest cut into. **THE NEXT DAY**.

I should point out that the fact that this whole thing was happening in the blink of an eye was indeed a blessing. No time for reflection. No time to be scared. No time even to reflect on what the final diagnosis might be.

BIOPSY BLUES

In fact, the only time I can truly say I was scared was when I was about to be sent down for the biopsy. The biopsy to discover what this shadow between my lungs was. Debbie was with me in the ward. We were partaking in our usual banter. The hospital porter approached. He smiled and took off the bed trolley brakes. He wheeled me away. Backwards. Debbie waved. A wave seemed eerie somehow. Fateful. A goodbye. Her silhouette got smaller and smaller as I dissolved into a mirage of nothingness.

My life had become a David Lean movie. Maurice Jarre's score was swelling in my head. Underscoring my life. I was no longer twenty-eight. I was five. Six at the most. I was wrapped in a blanket of uncontrollable fear. A fear that has no explanation or target. But just is. Fear.

*'Got to get off this trolley. Got to get off this trolley and run. And run. And run. And keep on running. And run and run and run and run and run. As far from here as possible. As far from **this** as possible. And run and run and run and run. HELP ME SOMEBODY!'*

I bit my lip to stop myself crying and I drew blood. Nothing compared to the slice that the surgeon was about to make into my skin and my insides, but real blood nonetheless.

The astoundingly instinctive and magical nurse walking with me to the operating theatre gently put her hand on my shoulder and, like an angel, just stroked me down from the heavens, away from hyperventilation and back on some sort of even keel.

The exceptionally posh anaesthetist numbed my arm and administered the first dose: *'This will feel like two glasses of claret... Now I want you to count backwards from five. This next injection will feel like eight glasses of claret.'*

'Five, four, three...' White. Out.

ME, MY CANCER AND I

In the period leading up to my diagnosis there was very little doubt that my pineapple head was a result of something growing inside me. That unavoidably led to the thought that if the men and women in their white coats or their blue ER scrubs couldn't stop the pineapple growing, then it would inevitably eventually explode. My head, that is. And leave a sticky pineapple mess. And a dead Raz.

I had already tried to imagine how a negative diagnosis might make me feel. I believed I would cope and be terrified in equal measure. However, it is fair to say that a vast part of me fully expected that being told I have an illness that had a decent chance of making me disappear would fill me up with such crippling, paralysing terror that I would spend my chemotherapy time curled in a foetal ball staring into a void of zeros. I say I expected that would be the case; the truth is I didn't know what to think.

I am walking around in a daze. I have an air of someone who's fine. Apart from my massive swollen neck. I can't stop to think about stuff. If I stop to think, I might just crumble. I have Jarvis Cocker in my ear telling me I'll never watch my life slide out of view. I am watching my life. I am also in it. It feels like I am translucent. They can see straight through me. I have no middle. Is this a daze? I think this must be fear. I think this must be what fear feels like? If this IS fear, why am I sort of euphoric at the same time? That seems just wrong.

Just as death is abstract, so is waiting for a diagnosis when, deep down, you are pretty damn sure of what the outcome will be. However hard you imagine it, it is still not real until the words come out of the doctor's mouth.

It's like England taking penalties against Germany. The whole thirty minutes of extra time is laced with the sinking feeling that a penalty shootout against the Germans inevitably means only one thing.

Lose. Lose. Lose.

And you're in a strange fucked-up haze of plurality. Because you are 100 per cent certain that you will not win. You are certain one of your players will sky the ball way over the crossbar. You are certain Germany will find the far corner of the net with pinpoint precision every single time.

You're not going to win. You know that.

In fact, you're going to lose. You know that.

You're doomed. You know that.

Yet, inside you, there's a stabbing, breathless pain.

It's **hope**. That old manipulator, **hope**.

And those two feelings sit alongside each other:

Hope and **absolute certainty of failure**.

The very combination of the two churns your stomach to cyclone proportions.

That's what it feels like waiting for the diagnosis.

Suspended – breathless – hopeful – agony.

THE RESULTS SHOW

Today was results day. On the one hand, I seemed to be dealing with this craziness pretty damn well – if I say so myself – and, on the other, I was perfectly able to just block it all out completely. To the point where I had actively chosen not to speculate as to what the pineapple-head biopsy may discover.

The previous night I had a gathering of people at my flat. What was meant to be a celebration of the day of my birth ended up as a show of support for me the day before my diagnosis. Conjecture as to the outcome was minimal. It mainly came out of my own inappropriate mouth and from a very blunt American friend, Polly.

'It's either benign, in which case you are going to have to have a major operation to get it out. Or it's malignant, in which case you are going to have to spend the next year in heavy duty treatment. Either way you're fucked.'

Fucked indeed.

So when the consultant, still in his blood-splattered scrubs, delivered the results, I was a bit more prepared for what might be to come. Well, I say prepared, I was still blessed with wilful ignorance, so when he gave his diagnosis I didn't really register what it was.

'He's a very ill young man, he has Hodgkin's Disease,' he said, talking to my mother, as if I was as old as the eight-year-old I felt in that moment. My mother understood what Hodgkin's Disease was. She was much more clued up than me. Through the haze of denial, I deciphered slowly what it meant. It meant Germany had indeed won on penalties again! It meant **Cancer**.

I made a call to my friend Tiggy who was staying at my flat to help me through this weird bit of the journey. *'We're in the hat business.'*

Denial over. I was **Cancer** out. And **Cancer** proud.

As it turns out I didn't have Hodgkin's Disease. What I actually had was non-Hodgkin's lymphoma. They are quite similar. They are both cancers of the lymph system. Don't ask me what the major differences are. In 1995, I had only just discovered that you could search for information on a computer and that it could help you with lots of questions you might need answers to. My brother produced a few pages that he had 'downloaded'. His words, not mine. I didn't really want to know too much detail. In fact, I was happier not knowing. All I did know was that non-Hodgkin's lymphoma was the least good of the two options to get.

ODDS

The consultant may have guessed that, alongside my newly attained status as a young man with cancer, I was also a gambler. The biggest clue being that I never asked about the science of my illness. All I wanted to know was:

'What are my odds?'

'What odds will you give me on survival?'

Well, turns out the odds were pretty good.

Unlike blackjack in a casino, they were stacked in my favour. Although consultants liked to remove themselves from the buzzers and bells of conjecture, when pushed I was given about a 70 to 80 per cent chance of survival (depending on which consultant I asked and how I phrased/loaded the question). That's pretty good odds. Odds any true gambler would swallow up.

I was told that it was very treatable – especially for someone relatively young – but if it came back, then I would pretty much be toast. That's not the technical term they used. Though it wasn't far off.

And so with my heart in my mouth and cancer in my body, the next phase of my life was about to begin.

JAR. SPERM. SPERM. JAR

I was twenty-eight.

In the blink of an eye, I had a doctor's appointment, an X-ray, a shadow between my lungs, and stage 4 cancer. I was about to have heavy duty chemo. The last thing I was thinking about was babies. But the clever people at the Royal Marsden Hospital had seen this all before. They had treated slightly bolshie, somewhat bewildered twenty-eight-year-olds before. They knew the routine.

'Heavy chemo can make you infertile so in cases such as this we suggest you go to the clinic and deposit some sperm... OK?'

'OK.'

'We will need to postpone your first chemotherapy session so that you can do this, but that shouldn't be a problem.'

Shouldn't be a problem for who? I had psyched myself up for my first chemo session. I was ready for my first chemo session. I mean, I wasn't ready for it but I was ready to embrace not being ready for it.

And now they wanted me to give sperm.

Now, normally I am pretty generous in my sperm giving. I give sperm freely, in fact. Freely, openly and generously. Yes, I am a generous sperm-giving kind of guy. However, my sperm isn't normally deposited into a bottle and then a bank. That's not the kind of deposit that I'm used to. But despite, at the time, having zero desire for a child, I was persuaded that it couldn't hurt to have some in reserve. Some sperm reserve. In case of a drought.

I needed to get on with it, though, as it was made clear to me that time was not on my side and the sooner I deposited, the sooner

I could get on with chemo. In other words, the quicker I pumped stuff out of my body, the quicker stuff could be pumped in!

Like all NHS things that need to be speedy, this was speedy. An appointment was made for 9 a.m. the next day.

15 JUNE 1995. 8.50 A.M.

I was in the waiting room of the Fertility Clinic at the Queen Charlotte Hospital. Bottle in hand. Ready to fill it up. Well, actually, not ready. At all. Under instructions to fill it up. Only forty-eight hours earlier I had been diagnosed with cancer. I was not exactly in 'fill the bottle' mode. And the bottle was small. The end of the bottle was narrow.

How can I...?

Will I spill...?

What if I miss, do I tip it back...?

Are they better swimmers than me? I hope so.

How long before they cease to be active?

Don't those mini-mes have cancer too?

Do I need both hands to...?

I honestly think those few minutes at the Queen Charlotte Hospital were about the most surreal of my whole illness. There were a thousand things floating around my head. These included:

Cancer

Life

Death

Death

Sex

Desire

Babies

Breakfast

Cancer sperm banks

Banks

Life
Life
Life
Life
The intangibility of death
The possibility of death
The likelihood of death
Death
Life
Life
Life
Bacon
Sperm
Sperm
Sperm
Eggs
Eggs
Bacon
Sperm

LOUD HEAD

It was 9.01 a.m. It was pretty quiet in the waiting room, but pretty fucking piercing in my head. The madness running around in there wasn't conducive to getting turned on enough to be able to fill a thimble let alone a bottle.

Do I have any dark fantasies in the recesses of my mind reserved for a rainy day? Do I? God, I hope so, because it's fucking pouring in here!

MY NUMBER'S UP

And so my number was called. Number one. I was number one. I was directed down the hallway, bottle in hand, to the first door on the right. A sign outside the door said 'Partners Welcome'. I was alone. Thank God. I opened the door. I was transported to a seedy bedsit in Paddington in the 1970s. Not that I ever frequented a seedy Paddington bedsit in the 1970s. I would have been under ten years old. That would have been weird. Even weirder than this. And this was pretty off the scale weird.

BROWN

I closed the door behind me. Directly in front of me there was a single bed with a brown sort of bobbly corduroy-type bedspread on it. The brown curtains were well and truly closed. There was actually muzak playing. I white-noised it in my head. I didn't want to hear any words. That would not help. So I didn't hear what was playing. Maybe it was themed. Maybe 'Be My Baby' or 'Papa Don't Preach' or 'Stairway To Heaven'. Maybe. I don't know. There was a small table next to the bed on which sat a glass of water, a box of tissues and a pile of well-thumbed 'magazines' – with some pages stuck together no doubt. Next to the small table was an empty wastepaper basket.

I placed the specimen bottle on the table and sat on the bed. I stared straight ahead. I waited for inspiration. And waited. And waited. I looked around the room. This must be what prison feels like. Come to think of it (or should it be, think to come for it?), the room did somewhat resemble a prison cell.

I thumbed through the top magazine. Cheryl, twenty-three, from Cleethorpes followed my gaze. She knew she could do nothing for me. The opposite, in fact. She was taunting me. *'Come and have a go if you think you're hard enough.'* I wasn't. I closed the magazine. Trite, one-dimensional, vapid nakedness has its place, but this was neither the time nor the place.

JUST FILL THE BOTTLE

I took the bottle and the matter in hand. I closed my eyes and dug deep into that well of dark fantasy. Thankfully, the well was not completely empty. It was just about accessible. It was a long way down and it took ages to reach, but whatever *was* there seemed to do the trick. To some degree. I even managed the procedure without any spillage. And that was the second relief of the day.

I had been instructed to fill the bottle and take it immediately to the lab to make sure they were good enough swimmers. Otherwise no point in storage. Never store dead swimmers in the fridge. Pointless. I took it to the hairy man in the white coat standing behind the counter. I think he was a scientist. He wasn't instructed in the art of bedside manner (I am pretty sure having him in the room with me while I was trying to fill the jar would not have helped. But, then, you never know.). I gave the bottle to the hairy scientist and he said:

'*Is that all?*'

IS THAT ALL??? That's not really what you wanted to hear after you'd just mounted Everest.

DOUBLE THE LOAD

Humiliation laced with anger laced with deep embarrassment is not a cocktail to be wished for. However, I am English:

I smiled.

I apologised.

I apologised again.

I apologised once again.

I think hairy scientist man realised he had been a bit brusque (you think!) as he then very gently explained that what I had produced was only about three months' worth of sperm. In layman's terms (that is me), that means that when trying to get a woman pregnant that would give us only three goes (one go a month). Hairy scientist man suggested that for it to be a worthwhile storage, I needed to double the load. Six goes is a fair crack of the whip to make a baby, apparently.

FORTY-EIGHT HOURS FOR REGENERATION

Hairy scientist man explained that I needed to leave forty-eight hours for 'regeneration'! This really is beginning to replicate one of the more surreal episodes of *Star Trek*. First series, of course.

So I left. I had to postpone my first chemo appointment. AGAIN.

They understood. Of course. They were the most understanding people I have ever met. And I mean that with absolutely no hint of irony whatsoever.

TAKE TWO

My next appointment at the fertility clinic was set for 11 a.m. That didn't hold any significance for me until I arrived. I realised that previously I had had the luxury of being first in line. As I sat there waiting for my turn, I watched a series of men go through the depository door before me, bottles in hand. My mind couldn't help imagining what they were doing in there. Well, not exactly. I *knew* what they were doing in there, I just couldn't get those images out of my head. And not in a good way, you understand. I couldn't help wondering why all these men were there. How many reasons could I think of for a man having to give sperm? Despite it being a good game to pass the time, it was in no way going to help me do what I was about to do.

The guy before me was a vast bear of a man wearing a shiny suit that seemed three times too small for him. It was impossible to get out of my head the noise this man might make on point of ejaculation.

A kind of high-pitched, self-satisfied squeal. *'Oooooooooaaa-aaaeeeeeeeee.'*

Not helpful. Not helpful. Not helpful.

My number was eventually called and I entered the all too familiar stale smelling fertility cell. No welcoming partner by my side. Just me, my bottle and the faint echo of a giant's screeching orgasm. That wasn't the only thing to remind me of him. Being about tenth in the queue that day meant that the wastepaper basket next to the table was overflowing with used tissues.

Dark fantasy, dark fantasy, fantasy. Come to me. Please. Please. I can't do this without you. Pleeeeeeeasssssse... Oh my, now that IS dark. Wow! How did I get there? Wow. Fucking wow! This is good.

I lost myself for a moment and it was working and it was really working and...

yes, get the bottle...

yes, no spillage...

yes, every month counts...

yes...

and yes...

and YES...

There it is.

A done deal. A ton of stuff in there. Wow. At least three months' worth. Hairy scientist man's going to be really pleased with me. Yep. Good job.

I added to the used tissue mountain, and took my bottle out to hairy scientist man. He didn't really say much this time. He nodded, took the bottle, checked my name, registered the said bottle and left. And that was it. I was free to go. So I did. Go.

I went from the fertility hospital straight to the cancer hospital for Chemo numero uno.

And on the Tube from Hammersmith to South Kensington, I got the fear for the first time. Well, the first time since the diagnosis anyway. Up till then I had been occupied in doing stuff. Now something was going to be done to me. Something to try to kill the invasion inside me. And that was a bit bloody scary. It was. And the fear took me by surprise. And stepping through the doors of the Royal Marsden Hospital felt like the opening sequence to my own gothic nightmare.

No turning back now.

It makes sense to me now why they were so adamant that I make a deposit before my treatment. The start of a process like this is daunting and disorienting. You need any security that life can give you. Having sperm in the bank was definitely a comfort. Still is. Back then it was a nod to the normal life I would one day hopefully get back. Today it feels like a beautiful, tangible living symbol. A symbol of a time when I was allowed just a little bit of control over my life and its future, at the very moment when everything around me seemed to be going off kilter. More than that, it is a simple but glorious indication that life goes on.

Even on a shelf in a fridge somewhere in Hammersmith.

DIAGNOSIS CANCER

As a word. As just a word, CANCER does sound quite sinister.
Say it out loud now.

C A N C E R

It's a very breathy word.
There's almost too much air inside it.

C A N C E R

Try different ways of delivering it.

C
A
N
C
E
R

See how it sounds and how those sounds make you feel.

C
  A
    N
      C
        E
         R

Sing it to the tune of 'Amazing Grace':

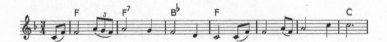

Can-cer, ca-a-ancer, can-cer, can-cer, can-cer ca-a-ancer, ca-an-CER

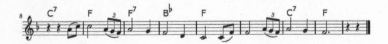

Can-cer, can-cer, can-cer, can-cer, can-cer ca-a-ancer can-cerrrrrrrrr

Creepy and glorious.

WARNING

If you are sitting on a bus reading this and obligingly following these instructions, be warned:

- If you are whispering it, you may sound like the 'cancer mouth bomber'. The Cancer Mouth Bomber is a strange evil loner with squinty eyes, wearing an eighties parka, who is often to be found on the top deck of the number 73 bus. The Cancer Mouth Bomber is endeavouring to infect the population by means of Cancer Whisper.
- If you are giving full vent to your lungs and shouting the word CANCER out loud and long, you will seem just plain scary and, before long, you will no doubt be arrested and removed by the cancer police.
- If you are singing it full pelt, like a hymn, you will just sound plain bonkers.

Regardless, it's one of those fantastic words that is so evocative and emotive that it is hard to know whether the actual form of the word or the letters within the word add to its power.

Let's say CANCER was called something different. Something softer with smoother vowels.

Shoop, maybe, or **shoom**.

Shoom. Yes. **SHOOM.**

Would that make a difference?

'What's wrong with me, Doctor?'

'Well, I am sorry to say you have stage 4 Shoom.'

Would that make things feel less deathly? Or soften the blow? Probably not. But it might help fewer people visibly wince when they hear the word.

For a while anyway. But it wouldn't last for long. The disease is such that any word would eventually take on the same iconic ugliness that pervades the word cancer. You can change the word but you can't change the illness. The only thing you have control of is how you respond to the diagnosis.

Diagnosis Shoom.

PART TWO:
THE TREATMENT

CANCER NEW

I loathe first days. Abhor them. First days at school or at work fill me up with paralysing, nausea-inducing dread. Every. Single. Time.

First day of chemo was like all first days rolled into one.

The Cancer Emperor of first days.

Everything was new.

This hospital was new. These doctors were new. Cancer was new.

And it wasn't fear that I was feeling. Not really. Just this immense new consciousness of being out of control. I hadn't yet learned the hospital/chemo/cancer routine. And I do like a routine. Until I have established a routine, there is no routine. And without routine I am in the deep end with no sodding armbands.

ROUTINES AND RITUALS

BC (Before Cancer), I had a whole phonebook of routines and rituals. I am not good with doubt. I like to know what I am eating, where I am going, who I am going with and who I'm going to meet there. I don't want to be surprised by an unanticipated visitor or an unexpected turn of events. I want to know what I know and know that that will in no way change.

So, entering this vast white chemo world with cancer under one arm and no routine under the other was not my idea of heaven. So to speak. What I needed was a few things to latch onto that would remind me of me. That would hopefully replenish me with some of the me that I had before this craziness began. And make me feel more equipped to cope.

The thing I needed most to make a routine out of a nightmare was to familiarise myself with my surroundings. To be comfortable in a building, I need to both know its architecture and be familiar with some of the people working within it. That is still the case today. When I work in a theatre for the first time it takes me a while to get the lie of the land. I know I have started to feel at home when I find myself confidently striding around tipping my head at people like some kind of nodding dog. So if you happen to have been in the Royal Marsden Hospital around the middle of June 1995, you may recall a strange, Jew-froed young man wandering seemingly aimlessly around the building trying to smile and make contact with as many people as possible. This may have been me trying hard to get to know my surroundings or someone altogether more sinister. Either way my advice would have been the same. Avoid at all costs.

I also discovered that I could trick myself into thinking hospital life was akin to home life by bringing with me a heap of stuff. Me stuff. Me stuff is ever-changing. By definition (mine), me stuff is just things that I surround myself with that put me at ease in an otherwise uneasy environment. Like my own personal comfort blanket of stuff! That doesn't make me eccentric at all. NOT AT ALL. Actually, you can't be eccentric if you know you're eccentric so that must mean I am totally normal. Totally. Anyway, my June 1995 stuff included:

- The new Nick Hornby novel – *High Fidelity*.
- A fake Sony Discman with Bruce Springsteen's *Greatest Hits* CD inside it (normally sacrilegious for a true Bruce fan to buy a greatest hits album but those commercially savvy record company types – aka 'money grabbing bastards' – cleverly added five new songs at the end of it to make it a 'must have' or a 'can't NOT have'.)

- A cutting from the *Guardian* on Arsenal's new 'unknown' signing Dennis Bergkamp.
- A copy of Terry Johnson's play 'Dead Funny' (no comment on my future prospects intended!)

Strangely, the one trait, above any other, that has always made me feel 'me' and has sat comfortably with me for as far back as I can remember is also something that I don't often actively think about. Can't think about. Until now. It's just in me. It's just me. Namely, the ability/desire to flirt. With just about anybody. In fact, I'll go so far as to say that flirting was and is an inalienable part of my identity. I have no idea why. I have no idea where the need comes from. I suspect it's linked, in some small way, to my addictive personality.

But looking back on it now, the more adept I became in the art of flirting, the more I was able to suppress the deeply shy little boy that lay large inside me. That discovery was huge to me. As a young boy/man my shyness often felt overwhelming and paralysing. So without really being conscious of it, flirting was a language that would help me navigate my way more comfortably through my life.

FLIRTATION COMFORT ZONE

By the ripe old age of twenty-eight I had become, so I thought, somewhat fluent in that ancient *lingua franca* of flirt and so, when I stepped through the doors of the Royal Marsden Hospital, it didn't take me long to notice that a fair proportion of the cancer nurses were young, attractive and, oddly, from New Zealand. I say oddly not because they were actually odd or because coming from New Zealand makes you odd, but because the Royal Marsden seemed to be swarming with men and women in nurses' uniforms from down under. An Antipodean nursing carnival.

Nurses have become my heroes. I will never, ever be able to find the right words to express how remarkable they were and are. Calm, patient, understanding and more caring than should be humanly possible. The nurses at the Marsden seemed unflappable. They also seemed flirtable with. Both the men and the women. Now, I have to point out that I knew I wasn't in a *Carry On* movie. These nurses were totally professional and dealt with a young man's desperate flirting, not by going behind the bike sheds or by delivering a bed bath de-arouser, but by giving enough back to feel like I wasn't being ignored but not enough to feel like I was getting somewhere. Story of my life! And it just meant that I didn't feel I was in the most alien place in the world. It meant that I could bring a tiny bit of me into my new environment. And a nurse's ability to recognise the needs of the individual is what sets them apart from mere mortals.

I can't say hospital ever felt like home. Or even felt like the norm. But sometimes it got quite close. And that felt good. And comforting. And that was pretty much all due to the brilliance of the nurses.

So with my routine sorted and my flirting possibilities identified, me and my illness set out on our journey together. Side by side, we climbed the emotional Pyrenees on our very own Tour de Cancer. I knew the mountainous journey ahead would often be gruelling, sometimes vicious, now and again heart-breaking, and once in a while sublime, but I would try very hard to steer away from second-guessing the future.

Tomorrow is tomorrow is tomorrow. As Shakespeare sort of said.

POV CANCER

Having cancer is kind of surreal. It feels like you are the narrator of your own cancer movie. The movie is from your point of view and the camera has been planted in your eyes. In this movie, you get to judge other people's reactions to you. The young man with cancer. You, the viewer, get to share that dark existence with him. The dark existence in his head in response to how someone reacts when he tells them he has the C word. Or CA word.

That is exactly how it felt. Being behind the lens and observing those around me, I tried really hard not to judge people. Because if you have expectations, they will inevitably lead only to disappointment. And that in turn will lead only to sadness. And that's exactly the kind of emotion you are working hard to stave off. Sadness in this context feels a little bit like self-pity, and self-pity can fuck right off right now.

I am trying to avoid any feelings that are implosive. That is to say any emotions that eat away at my insides. After all, there's a twelve-course tasting banquet going on inside me right now and I need to leave room for the James Bond of chemicals to kick the shit out of my unwanted guests.

CANCER HOTLINE

So I knew I must be open. I must be inclusive. I must fake it when I don't feel it. I must welcome you into my cancer world with open arms. Big Jewish open arms. Topol would have been proud! Word spread very quickly and the phone started to ring non-stop. And I answered thus:

'*Hello, Cancer Hotline.*'

Some people didn't react well to this greeting. It made them feel uncomfortable. My mother didn't like it at all. Or my cancer jokes. Why would she? The parent losing a child thing is so unimaginable that you don't want to be constantly reminded of the possibility by your warped youngest child.

'*Read all about it. Youngest child has cancer. Youngest child riddled with cancer.*'

And some people *are* going to feel uncomfortable and some people *are* going to back off, but as much as I could in some way create an environment that induced the people I wanted around me to **stay** around me, I couldn't single-handedly save some people from their own fears. And so I guess part of my – albeit subconscious – reasoning for being so openly '*Cancer, Cancer, I have Cancer*' was to intensify this moment in order to uncover the people who stayed and the people who ran. And it wasn't/isn't a judgement on the runners. It was much more to do with my desire to surround myself with people who enjoyed the me that I was at that moment rather than the me they needed me to be.

I didn't want people around me who were going to look at me and see my death.

I didn't want people around me who were going to look at me and see their death.

I just wanted people around me who were going to look at me and see **me**.

UNCONSCIOUS AVOIDANCE

And people did back off and that's totally OK. I am not sure they even knew that they were doing it. They were victim to it like I was victim to it. Their implosion was not conscious. In their head they were there for me. The fact that they hadn't said that or, indeed, hadn't said anything at all has never occurred to them. It's unconscious avoidance. And it's hard, real-life stuff. And it is sad. And it is painful.

But, hell, if we were all normal functional human beings, the world would be as dull as shit.

And if I were to confront them about it – those 'backer-offers' – I think they'd be mortified. They'd get that cold-sweat-down-the-back-of-the-neck feeling that a director gets when he puts his work in front of an audience for the first time and realises he's made a glaring error. They'd suddenly see themselves and the truth with crystal clarity and they'd feel like death. And I didn't need any competition in that department, thank you.

FRONT-ROW SEAT

Having a front-row seat to people's reactions was a luxury. It was the most fascinating and unique part of this whole illness thing. It was also almost an art form. Fantastic manipulation training for being a theatre director.

Directing is all about getting to know someone and then working out how to get the best out of them. The moment you start treating everyone in one uniform, blanket way, your number's up. You will end up with something bland, generic and expressionless.

It's the same in the theatre of cancer.

You must decide:

a. who you want accompanying you on this journey
b. how you want those people to feel and behave on that journey.

Once you have figured that out, you go into manipulation mode.

It is my job to set up the environment that would best allow those people that I want here with me to feel as comfortable as possible.

That's the point I think that some people forget.

You are the most powerful person in that room. **You** have the cancer. **You** are the elephant. So if **you** aren't comfortable, nor will they be. **You** have the power, so **you** have to set up the right environment.

It often comes as a real surprise the way people react. Sometimes their reaction can be wondrous and delightful, and at other times it can be terribly disappointing. The trick really *is* to try to 'treat those two impostors just the same'. But I can't deny it. Withholding resentment when you are already straining not to feel sorry for yourself can be really hard.

But we have to be better than that. Bigger than that. Because, like I keep saying, **we** have the power, not them.

This is my movie and if I want to get good, relaxed performances out of my co-stars, I need to create the perfect setting for that to happen.

MY CAMERA

My camera sees people in extreme close-up.

People looking at me, looking at them, looking at me.

My camera captures in tiny detail their reaction the first time they see me.

Do I look the way they expected me to look? Do I look worse or better?

However brave a face you care to show the world, hidden beneath the bravado is a child. A lonely, wide-eyed child who wants to run and keep on running. You know you can't. You know you have a duty, not to yourself, but to the people who believe that you are strong, and that the strength of your personality will pull you through the hell. So you don't run but you sure as hell want to.

In extreme close-up I am able to see exactly how much effort that particular person is putting into this moment in order to make themselves seem relaxed in my presence. And people do put so much effort into controlling their facial expressions. They think I can't see how uncomfortable they are. The amount of effort they are putting in is both beautiful and heart-breaking.

I am able to adjust my face to theirs, my body language to theirs, until they eventually loosen up, drop their façade and be the person I want to visit me rather than the person they think I want them to be.

It's a complex movie that needs more than one viewing to understand it.

It's a movie that tries to get under the skin of a cancer patient's visitors.

CANCER CAMERA

The cancer camera can see through any membrane. It can pinpoint rare emotional responses. It cannot be purchased. It is unique to you and is guaranteed to make you an award-winning director.

The cancer camera not only shines the light on those who have been kind enough to come and see you, it also affords you an opportunity to not be you. For a moment at least:

- I am De Niro in an early Scorsese movie. I am more aggressive than I need to be and my visitors are not comfortable at all. *'Are you looking at me?'*
- I am in a 1970s disaster movie. I am Paul Newman. I have cancer but even so I am still the one leading everyone out of the burning building. I am the stunningly good-looking one who risks his life to save the world. And I play pool and I don't sweat.

- I am Bill Murray in *Cancerbusters*. I slay cancer. Mine and everyone else's. I do it on the back foot with a twinkle in my eye. I am the wittiest man alive and my one-liners are to die for!
- I am Hugh Grant in a Richard Curtis movie and everybody is reciting famous poems by my bed and weeping. And Rowan Atkinson is a vicar about to read me the last rites. And it's all a bit awkward when he realises I'm a Jew. And we all laugh and weep and it rains but nobody notices.

I was me. Still am.

I fall asleep.

You, my visitor, are still there when I wake up. That's nice.

My camera keeps running.

Nobody shouts, '*Cut.*'

There will be no wrap party. For a while anyway.

WHY ME? WHY NOT ME?

Every day I would wake up and for just a split second, I would think: *I may be cancer-free. It may have disappeared or it may have all been one long Bobby Ewing dream.*

But then reality would bite and I'd realise that this wasn't a soap opera. Not a tele-visual one anyway. It was what some people call real life.

*And I **do** have cancer.*

*And I **am** going to have to 'battle' again today.*

And when you're feeling like shit and you have that taste in your mouth that's like a cross between a rusty spoon and mild cow dung, and you are too tired to sit up, let alone get out of bed, it's very easy to cry inwardly, *'WHY ME?'*

Inward crying is less embarrassing than outward crying. Though outward crying may be more cleansing. In fact, it's the new thing. Tantrum yoga it's called. It's designed to have you breathe, dance and scream your way to better health. I kid you not. You can get DVDs on it and everything!

Let's try it now:

*'WHY ME? WHY GIVE **ME** CANCER AND NOT THAT CREEPY ANNOYING STARING MORON OVER THERE STARING AT MY BALD FUCKING HEAD. WHY? WHY? WHY ME?'*

Shit, that was a bit loud. The creepy annoying staring moron doesn't look creepy at all. Or a moron. He just looks scared. Of me.

Anyway, how helpful is *'WHY ME?'*?

I don't see how *'WHY ME?'* gets you anywhere at all. Not

only is it completely energy sapping but it is also pointless. Totally pointless.

You *do* have cancer.

FACT.

Pondering on *why* you have it and whether someone pointed their big lottery finger and chose you is not only irrelevant and ridiculous but it will also eat away at your insides. And you already have that going on.

'Why **Not** Me?' is:

- Much more fun.
- Much more empowering.
- Much more ego-fuelled and unique-making. After all, one in three people get cancer at some point in their lives. You don't want to be left out.

'Why **Not** Me?' is also a much more revealing and rewarding conceit.

Without the insufferable notion of 'be positive', 'Why **Not** Me?' injects you with *positivity by stealth*.

It also alleviates some guilt as you become the hero who saved someone else from that same fate.

I took one for the team. The cancer team.

Or should I say the '*I don't have cancer, never will have cancer*' team.

If only they knew, they would hold me aloft on their shoulders. Their shoulders that lead to heads with hair on them.

- *They would call me a hero.*
- *A prince among all men.*
- *Albeit a prince with an illness.*
- *But a prince nonetheless.*

- *I don't graduate to King unless I...*
- *Well, anyway, Prince will do.*

And 'Why **Not** Me?' is also so much more than that.

It's a celebration of the lottery of life. It's actually an affirmation of me. Of my propensity to be able to cope with this mystery inside me.

'Why **Not** Me?' is my *all-knowing-imaginary-so-called-superior-being* and it is saying:

'*Hmm... let's choose Raz, he has the capacity, the personality and the soul to deal with this major life-threatening illness; he has the strength of character to "enjoy" the multiple challenges this illness will set him and he will face it head on.*'

'Why **Not** Me?' should make you smile, should make you proud, make you feel unique, make you want to share it with your friends and glory in the insight it gives you.

And that never goes away.

It has lived with me every day for the last twenty-two years and it is here now.

It is the very reason why I want to share that insight with you.

The very thing that propels me forward even on those days when doors keep slamming against my soul.

WHY NOT ME?

THIS TOO SHALL PASS

Having cancer puts you into a world of unknowns, intangibles and the indefinable. It puts you into a world that to some degree you have no control over. It leaves you at the mercy of white cells inside you and white coats around you. For evil or for good, it's out of your hands. However strong you are, however well you seem to be dealing with it all, you really can't do it alone. And even if you are surrounded by a mountain of supporters, well-wishers and carers, sometimes you feel a loneliness that is unlike any you have ever experienced.

It is like being trapped, on your hands and knees, in a hole in the ground. You can feel the walls very slowly closing in around you. You can't *see* them closing in because it's pitch dark but you can *feel* them and you know you have to get out of there. You know you have to get out of there but you are on your hands and knees and you can't even remember how to crawl. You have lost all sense of your own humanity. Lost all awareness or understanding of how this human that is you behaves, thinks or moves. You have even lost the rational thought mechanism that would allow you to understand that you *have* to escape before the walls choke you to death. If you had rational thought right now, that would surely trigger your brain to remind you how to physically move, which in turn might enable you at least to make an attempt to get the fuck out of this hole. And even if you could do that, you wouldn't even begin to know where to go. There is a tiny taunting speck of white in the distance but it never stays still long enough for you to realise that heading for it is your ticket out of there. And there are millions of people around you, but you have no concept or desire to communicate with them. Because you know they can't help you right now. You know that the only person who can help you now is you.

And you are no help at all.

And this is isolation right here. This is what true loneliness is. And at times like this you just have to ride it out because it will pass. When and how and why, you have no clue. But it will. Pass.

HUG THE TUMOUR

The hardest thing to explain to anybody is how it makes you feel to know that the cancer is inside you. Has invaded you. For me, as I've said, it was never a 'why me?' thing. But it *was* a thing. Inside me. Inside ME. And its presence was weird and invasive and intrusive. And its presence didn't upset me, it just annoyed the fuck out of me. Because I don't like hanging out with big crowds of people at the best of times. Plus, I'm a control freak. So an ad hoc party at my house with a gallon of gate-crashers is my kind of hell. But you get used to it. You do. And you learn to embrace it, and them, to some degree. Or at least I did. Embrace them.

And that was hard for me, but hopefully harder for them. If my tumour was anything like me, it wouldn't have liked to be touched, let alone embraced.

I like the idea that, just to annoy it, you might give it a big old smothering hug now and again. The tumour doesn't know what to do with this hug. It feels like a spotty, excruciatingly embarrassed teenager when his mum kisses him in front of his friends and wipes his face with a licked handkerchief. Maybe embarrassing the tumour in front of its friends will make it shrink. So it retreats to its room to play loud grunge music. And pick its spots. And do other stuff to its teenage self. And disappear. Hopefully. And you can get back to your retreat in Other Land.

OTHER IS

Other is something to do with not quite being part of the norm, part of the mainstream, part of the gang. Other can be enforced upon you or embraced by you. In my case it is/was both. Other surrounded me. It surrounded me because for some reason the alternative – normality – never really offered itself to me. I tried to push 'other' away. In the act of trying and failing, I realised that it was a brilliant mask behind which to hide. Eventually I learned to love it and now I find it almost impossible to ascertain which is the mask and which is the me. Either way it is me.

At twenty-eight, that mask became a really vital part of my stay-alive toolkit. I could present a face to the world at the same time as trying to shield myself and my soul from the darkness that I might be retreating to. Sneaky. Handy. Not always that healthy.

Emotionally speaking, that is.

SEX AND CANCER, PART ONE – IBETTERFUCKHIMJUSTINCASEHEDIES

Sex. Cancer.

Two words that scare the fuck out of a lot of people. Individually.

Put them together and we're in a world of pain.

Or beauty. Or pain. Or painful beauty. Or beautiful pain.

Sexy cancer. Cancerous sex.

When you have cancer, what you're looking for is blood that will give you life. Lifeblood. You're also looking for things that will make you feel sort of normal and real and alive. Sex ticks those boxes. For me at least.

Sex has been my language of choice for as far back as I can dare to imagine.

The language of love, is a strange indecipherable over-analysed thing. I have always been sceptic number one when it comes to true expressions and demonstrations of love and affection. They are rare. The Facebook world has ruined us. Almost all love declarations now seem to be easy, trite and without thought. I want to live in a *Brief Encounter* world where love expressions cost much. Where they constantly battle against an ingrained reserve. Where expressions of love are so hard won that the tiniest look can make your heart sing like Mario Lanza.

The language of love, I struggle with. The language of sex, I don't. It's a much more immediate and tangible form of expression. It's a language I have spent my whole life learning. It's a language through which I am able to share more of myself than in any other mode of expression. It's a cocoon in which I can become someone else. An open, sensitive, affectionate someone. It works best when it is adrenaline-fuelled. Which is always good for an addict! From a very early age, I was aware that this was something exciting, something unique, something I could own. A medium of communication like no other.

Cancer leaves you bereft. Way outside your zone of comfort. It strips you of all that you thought you had. All that you thought you knew. Turns you into a child again. A child with little education because he has lost most of it in the flood. The cancer flood. In my desperate struggle to stay afloat, I searched for something, anything, that would make me feel like me again.

Sex was that thing.

I instinctively knew I had to take myself through my own backstory and try to reposition that old sexual confidence into the heart of cancer-riddled me. If I could remember and almost relearn some of that confidence and combine it with my newly found cancer swagger, I might be on to something.

And it seemed to work. As I relived my sexual history in my mind, every memory reminded me a little more of my true place in the world. Every memory injected a bit more fuel into me. Every memory normalised me just a little more. Until eventually I had rediscovered some of my fluency and was confident enough to put it into practice.

And that was a big key for me. Rediscovering myself through reliving key moments of my past. By putting all those pieces together, I felt nearly whole again, nearly normal, nearly me. Nearly.

VIRGIN RAZ

I reached puberty at the relatively early age of eleven and from then on I was desperate to discover the hidden secrets of sex. That need, that desire, that throbbing urge wasn't helped by having two older brothers who would talk about their conquests all the time and who took delight in constantly drawing attention to the doughty sword of virginity hanging over my head.

A typical dinner conversation:

'*Have you done it yet? Have you? Well, have you? Have you?*'

'*Have you? Have you? Have you?*'

'*You done it yet? Have you? Have you? Have you?*'

At **twelve** years old, I would just laugh.

At **thirteen**, I would go bright red, die inside and laugh.

At **fourteen**, I would just stare in horror, make some squealing noise that was meant to signify a yes but had *NO NO NO, OF COURSE NOT, NO NO NO* written all over it.

'*Have you done it yet? You popped your cherry yet? Done it?*'

At **fifteen**, I would not laugh. I would say '*Fuck you, it's none of your business.*'

'*Come on. You lost it yet? Got your leg over?*'

At **sixteen**, I would say nothing and feel nothing.

'*Well? Well? Have you? Have you still got your V plates? Have you parked the pink Porsche down the side alley yet?*'

At **seventeen**, I would say yes. It was a lie.

'*Come ON! Have you done the dirty yet? Have you? Have you?*'

At **eighteen**, I would say yes. It wasn't a lie.

And what a relief it was to not have to lie. Thirty-seven seconds of relief on the kitchen floor with Rachel Channing, to be precise!

Along the teenage way, I tried to play out my sexual urges like a weird early eighties movie. In my memory I saw a boy who was filled with an extraordinary mix of blind panic and innate confidence when it came to all matters of sex. The panic was partly just the usual sexual panic of youth but it was also a reaction to the strange sexual arrogance that I knew also existed inside me. The young me was panicked because he wondered whether all the sexual greatness that he had to offer would ever be received by anyone ever. He really did feel that! If the twenty-eight-year-old me could just rediscover a tiny bit of that bizarre arrogance, he might be on to something. If the twenty-eight-year-old me could remind himself of a time when hope and delusion were fuelled by innocence rather than desperation, his present predicament might look a little different.

I was lying on a bed in the day clinic ready to have my first wrestle with chemo. I wasn't prepared for it. I wasn't ready for it. I didn't want it. It said on the chart at the end of my bed that I was twenty-eight years old. I was not. I was eight. Nine at most! I was a child. And all this was just plain odd. Everything and everyone seemed the size of a house. And I was the size of a gnat. That's what it felt like to be me. When I was eight, I wanted to be eleven. Eleven would be proper. Would be old. Would be proper old. Eleven would be playground superior.

I lay on a bed in the day clinic and I yearned to be eleven again. Longed for it.

Take me back there. To eleven. Please. Let's go. I want to be big again. I want to be on the edge of grown up. Not the gnat puerile nothing I am now.

THE DELUSIONS OF YOUTH

I am eleven years old. I am helping Miss Harrison put the music stuff away. The drums always go in last. The drums live in the top cupboard. The routine is always the same. Miss Harrison would climb on the table and I would hand the drums to her. This was our routine. IS our routine. I watch her climb onto the table. I feel the thrill inside me when she stands on her tippy toes to reach the top cupboard and her long slender calf muscles extend to the max. I know she is doing this for my benefit. I don't quite know what this is, but I think the adults call it flirting. Yes, she is flirting with me. Definitely. I can't control my breathing. Can't control anything! I know she is about to climb down *off the table, take my almost spot-free face in her hands (thank God I applied my zit cream this morning) and kiss me and kiss me and kiss me. And she will be the one. The one who... And she does climb off the table but she doesn't take my face in her hands. Which is strange. She must be waiting for the perfect moment. Or maybe she is shy. That's really sweet. Endearing. Maybe she's waiting for me to make the move? Maybe I should. Maybe I should just kiss her. I know that's what she wants. Maybe I need to just kiss her to let her know that I am OK with the age gap. Am fine with it. Am totally OK that she's really old. That's what she wants me to do. She wants me to put her at her ease and kiss her. She is nervous because it means so much to her and she is shy and she wants me to make the first move and she wants me to hold her face in my hands and kiss her and then she can relax and just run with it. The way she has in her dreams for weeks and weeks. The way we both have. And maybe this is HER first time too and maybe we can both just get lost in each other's first time. And I can tell her not to worry, that I know what to do. That I have two older brothers who have done it. 'I know what to do. Don't worry, Shirley (that was Miss Harrison's first name so I think she'd like me to use it. It would thrill her). Don't worry, Shirley, I know what to do. I have two older brothers who have done it.' And we will be together and we **will** do it. And I will be able to sit at the dinner table and boast about my girlfriend, Miss Harrison. Shirley. And I wouldn't have to lie. And Shirley would come over for dinner and eat with us. Come to think of it, scrap that. I think it would be a bit awkward for my family. They don't know anything about music. No. This will be our thing. And we will decide between us when we want to make it public. When we want to declare our love to the world. And so she comes down from the table. Looking like a goddess, may I add. And I know that I have to make that move. I know she is desperate for me to do it. Desperate for me to take twenty-something her in my eleven-year-old arms and kiss her. When shall I do it? Now? Yes? Yes. I have seen it on telly. On* The Sweeney. *I will just walk up to her. Look up. Look her in the* *eyes. She will bend down towards me and when she gets close enough I will reach out my arms and softly grab the back of her neck and pull her towards my virtually zit-free face. Thank God I brushed my teeth this morning. I am going to do it. I take a deep breath and slowly walk towards her. Just at that moment, my mother arrives. I can see the disappointment in her face. Miss Harrison's, not my mother's.*

I can tell that her 'Thanks for the help, Darren' was really 'Next time. Next time we will truly consummate the burning passion that is most clearly between us.'

But next time never came. Thankfully for her. But the delusional eleven-year-old always believed that it might.

Maybe Shirley Harrison is out there now ruminating on the what ifs.

'What if the eleven-year-old Darren Shaw had taken me in his arms and kissed me all those years ago. Life might have been so so different!'

Ain't that the truth!

And I lay there, in the day patient clinic, watching peculiar coloured chemicals about to be pumped into me, smiling at the thought of that absurd eleven-year-old. Twenty-eight was proud of eleven. Fifty is, too. Proud that he could dare to want to be different. Proud that he wasn't ashamed of that difference. And that memory and that pride made my childlike fears begin to dissipate. The syringe looked almost normal size. It looked bearable. I watched as the first flow of chemicals was pumped through the cannula into my veins. I was shocked at how cold it felt as it hit my blood. It wasn't painful shock. Just cold shock. I closed my eyes in avoidance. I needed more weird-child me. More adult-child-adult me.

STALKER ME

I am twelve years old. I am on the Tube. I see a woman. She is really, really old and really, really sexy. She is off-the-scale old. Probably about twenty-one. I know! Old as life. There is something beyond the old that magnetically draws me to her. She is without a doubt the sexiest woman I have seen since Miss Harrison. And I do know what sexy means. Sexy means that my heart starts to beat out of control fast and I go hard. Simple as that. I don't go hard, my penis does. And this woman does both to me. The heart thing and the hard thing, and I am compelled to follow her. I'm not sure what I will do beyond that. Haven't thought that far ahead. But it's fine. I'll deal with it. I'm Darren Shaw. I can deal with stuff. Plus I'm sure women are OK with twelve-year-old boys following them. Totally. And she does seem to be OK with it because after a twisty follow around the Tube station, she asks me my name. She is twenty-one. Probably. I am twelve. Definitely.

'My name's Eleanor. What's yours?'

She has a strange foreign sounding accent. With a deep squeal I tell her.

'Darren. Darren Shaw.'

We get to the platform and she puts her arm round me. We are sitting on the platform seat thing. She offers me a cigarette. I suavely decline. She puts her arm round me again. I didn't know what freezing was till this moment. I freeze. Her arm draped around my shoulder is the most uncomfortable sensation I have yet felt in my vast twelve years of life. And when I said freeze, what I should have said is that every single bit of me freezes except one tiny bit of me, which had been frozen solid, but now defrosts into a lifeless lump of unused flesh. And the Tube arrives and she gets up and jumps on board. She turns and looks at me. I am stuck on the platform not knowing what to do. She is beckoning me to join her but my feet won't move. I look at my watch and it is five already and I have to be home for supper by six and if I get on the Tube with her I will be late and how will I explain that to my mother and my mum's a bit scary when she's angry like the time she washed my mouth out with actual soap and water when I told her to fuck off and the doors slowly close and my feet are still glued to the platform and the train slowly moves off. And Eleanor keeps my gaze *the whole time. And the whole time she is wearing a sly grin as if to say, 'That showed you, kid. That showed you not to follow a strange woman double your age. Live and learn.'*

And I stand there and stand there and stand there. I feel the flush of youthful guilt fill up my cheeks. And I have lived and I definitely have learnt. I have. I know that I won't follow a woman again. Not till I am much much older anyway!

And my mind jolted back into the reality of chemo land. I was more than a little bit impressed by the strength of purpose of that twelve-year-old. So much need and adrenaline in someone so young. If I could just have 30 per cent of that adrenaline back. Forty maybe. If I could have some of his energy and focus and drive and youthful lust, I may kick this thing sooner rather than later. I may even have an amazing ride along the way. So to speak.

The nurse patted me on the hand.

'All done,' she said. 'If you just lie here for a few minutes while we do the chart and stuff, then you can be on your way.'

I was OK until that moment. The re-programming had been going swimmingly. The memory of the confidence of my youth had got me this far without too much fuss. But something was different. I knew I would walk out of there a changed man. Changed because there was no escape now.

I have cancer. I am having chemo. I have had my first chemo. This is real. Life. No escape.

Dread began to creep up on me. Dread of all this. Dread of the real world. Dread of the future. Dread of now. I close my eyes and desperately *Doctor Who* myself back fifteen years.

THE FULL HOUR OR JUST THE HALF?

I am fourteen years old. I have lived through three years of no-sex purgatory and I am ready to do something about it. Be more proactive about it. I know where my father keeps his magazines. We all know where my father keeps his magazines. In the back of those magazines, there are adverts. For all sorts of things. Most of which baffle me. What is a sex toy anyway? And why are they advertising toys in a magazine that is clearly meant for grown-ups? But I do know what a visiting topless massage is. I do. And I know that they often do more than just massages. They do. How do I know that? I am not so sure. I have older brothers. That must be it. So I spend three months saving every penny I can. Down the back of the sofa there is always cash. Sometimes the biggest coin, the fifty pence coin, would be lodged deep under the cushions. Finding one of those is like Arsenal winning the FA Cup. That happened last year. Arsenal beat Man U and my hero Liam Brady was the Man of the Match. I have finally collected enough money. I'm sure she won't mind bags and bags of coins. Money is money, right? I wait till two in the afternoon on a summer holiday Tuesday because I know nobody will be home for three hours. I pick up the phone and dial the number.

'Hello.'

'Er, hello.'

'Can I help you?'

'Is this the, erm, visiting massage service?'

'Yes, it is.'

'Can I book, erm, a visiting massage?'

'Certainly, sir. Can I just check that you are over eighteen?'

'Oh yes. Yes. Yes.'

'Good. We have to check, you understand.'

'Oh yes. Yes. Yes. Of course.'

'Would you like the full hour or just the half?'

'The what?'

'The full hour or just the half?'

'Um… um. Oh. OH! Erm. The. Erm. The. Erm. Half of the hour. I mean, half an hour please. Thank you.'

'Certainly. sir. The fee will be thirty pounds plus the taxi fare.

Cash on arrival. Would you like that immediately?'

'Erm. YES. I mean, yes. Thank you.'

'Certainly, sir, and what is your address?'

'Erm, 4, Oak… Erm, can I just ask. Erm, do you do, erm, erm, erm, erm, erm, extras?'

'Erm, extras, sir?'

'Erm, yes. Erm, you know. Erm. Err… Extras. Do you do erm… erm… extras?'

'Anything beyond our normal service you will have to discuss with the masseur when she arrives, sir.'

'OK.'

And I give my address and book the 'topless visiting massage'. And I get off the phone and my heart is out of my chest and breathing is a problem. I walk around the room in a circle for ages. Yes. Yes. Yes. I can't breathe. I can't breathe. I can't breathe. And breathless excitement slowly turns to breathless panic.

*What am I doing? She's going to come here. Actually going to come here. And I will have to get naked for her. I will have to do naked. For her. With her. I may be a touch out of my depth here. Maybe. Even me. Even I. Maybe. NO! I can do this. Can I? Yes. Of course. But I **am** only fourteen. I don't need to rush this. I am only fourteen. I am not the adult I think I should be. I am only fourteen and my virginal sexual urges have pushed me into unthinkingly doing something that I am not ready for. I am not ready for this. Not ready. Not ready. Not ready. When I say not ready, what I actually mean is I am ready but not now. Now is not when I am ready. I pick up the phone and even more hesitatingly cancel the 'massage'. Relief invades every bit of me. I can breathe again.*

As I lay there, in the day patient clinic, waiting to be discharged, I smiled at fourteen's lucky escape. He was spiralling groin first towards adulthood, and just at the last minute he had the insight to save a little bit of his innocence for a rainy day. And once he made that phone call he could breathe easier. For a while anyway. Fourteen years later, that was all I was looking to do. To breathe. To find a bit of the old me, make a new me and breathe. And the memories puffed me up and propelled me out of the hospital front door and readied me for what was to come.

Looking back on all this from behind the computer screen, I am so proud of twenty-eight in that moment. I am proud of eleven, twelve and fourteen too. Twenty-eight instinctively knew that to get through some of the big stuff, he had to find the thing about himself that made him feel special. Unique even. He found that in the extraordinary sexual confidence of eleven and twelve and the eventual self-awareness of fourteen. When I left the hospital that day, I *did* leave with a swagger. But the swagger wasn't about sex, it had just been triggered by its memory. The swagger was about an innate understanding that I was probably going to be OK. At least for today anyway. But cancer swaggers don't last too long when you're a gambling addict. No. My swagger soon tuned into a slightly panicked shuffle. A shuffle that took me straight from the Royal Marsden Hospital in South Kensington to Napoleons Casino in Leicester Square.

CANCER VERSUS GAMBLING, PART ONE

- Cancer is an insidious disease that is all-consuming, eats away at your insides and occupies your mind and your soul at every waking and sometimes sleeping moment.
- Gambling addiction is an insidious disease that is all-consuming, eats away at your insides and occupies your mind and your soul at every waking and sometimes sleeping moment.

I've told you how gambling came into my life from an early age. From the eleven-year-old's winning adventure at the dog track to the twelve-year-old's Vegas wonderland to the Edinburgh student's Chinese buffet casino residence, and on.

What I now know is that there was a cavernous hole deep inside me that ached to be filled. Along the way to my fifty years of life so far, I have tried to fill that hole countless times and with countless things. And gambling filled that hole. And cancer widened that hole and filled that hole. And gambling filled the hole that cancer had widened.

Gambling was a devourer of time. Seven hours sitting at a blackjack table felt like a few minutes. The world as I knew it disappeared. I was gripped by its hypnotic claw. I couldn't move. Didn't move. Didn't need to move. Didn't want to move. All of the day's appointments went for nothing because I couldn't leave. I couldn't leave if I was winning because I may have been on a streak. I couldn't leave if I was losing because I was definitely, definitely going to win it all back. Definitely.

And that's the decaying thing about being a gambling addict. Your level of certainty is heaven high. Your next bet is the one that will take you back on top. Take you to your diamond-encrusted floating paradisiacal nirvana. So it'd be stupid to stop now. Criminal even.

BACK IN THE ROOM

On 13 June 1995, I was diagnosed with cancer.

On 14 June 1995, I was at my usual blackjack table in Napoleons Casino, Leicester Square. I was in shock from the diagnosis and pain from the biopsy. Blackjack focus was my unmatchable numbing remedy. I climbed back into my focus bubble. I shut out the world around me. I was never the most sociable gambler at the best of times. Gambling wasn't a sharing thing. Gambling was pure self. I wanted to get lost in it. Not chat about it.

FILTH

Gambling addiction is mental filth. You know you should stop but you can't. You know that you shouldn't be thrilled when you lose but you sort of are. You are a millefeuille of self-hatred and this is your fuel. And if you talk to anyone else while you are doing it, you might just have to admit that this is awful, that this is wrong. If you start admitting that, then ultimately you might have to stop. Gambling. And you absolutely don't want to do that. Absolutely not. You need to stop. But you don't want to. So at the best of times I didn't speak to anyone. I was in a miasma of bewilderment. I have no idea if I lost or I won. I suspect I may have won. Don't know why. Beginner's luck perhaps. A beginner of cancer, that is. Not gambling.

CHEMO DAYS

It's hard to try to capture the bizarre, light-headed, sick-in-your-mouth empty feeling that was having chemotherapy. The night before always felt like the Sunday before school. All I ever wanted to do was run. Away. But I forced myself to stay and fight. It's even harder to capture that feeling in the past tense so we are going back to the now that is almost every Thursday from the second half of June 1995. This particular time is about six weeks into my treatment. As you will see, things weren't going well.

A THURSDAY IN THE SECOND HALF OF JUNE 1995. LONDON

Today is chemo day. I slept well last night. Like a child on Christmas Eve. Excited about going to sleep in order to wake up to get his presents but with a knotted feeling of fear about the possibility of his presents being shit. Although I am not sure a seven-year-old would have quite so much insight about his inner psychological make-up.

Today is chemo day. I try to open my eyes but they seem to be glued together. As I wrestle with my eyelids, I notice that I can't really breathe. I have a granite bowling ball lodged in the back of my throat forcing down on me every time I try to open my larynx. My skin feels like it has turned itself inside out. My body is ganging up on me. I am lying in an Olympic pool of sweat.

Today is chemo day. I might just lie here quite still forever. If I don't move, try not to breathe and don't try to open my eyes, all this might disappear. All this might disappear. All this. Not just this. This now. But all this. And I have been dealing really well with all this.

I have made countless bad cancer jokes about all this.

I have had lots of hats bought for me, to cover the side effects of all this.

I have continually stuck two fingers up at all this.

All this was a fucking breeze. Was. All this.

Until all this.

Today is chemo day. As I lie here motionless, my heart is beating out of my chest. I know that all this is just the beginning. I know that the road ahead is way longer than I will allow myself to imagine. After all, I have closed myself off from the truth by presenting to the world an image of a man who is really open about his recent hard-core diagnosis. A man who is inclusive and who doesn't seem to take it too seriously. That is my escape route. And it isn't an entirely truthful one.

Today is chemo day. As I lie here motionless, my whole body sweats and shakes in equal measure. I may as well have stepped onto a landmine. There is no escape from the reality of all this. I can't face today. Today can bugger off. I am going to disappear under my duvet and watch the OJ trial. Simpson that is, not orange juice. Orange juice is not on trial. Yet. Though if it were, I'm sure its defence would be pithy! See, even my shit jokes can't shake me out of my darkness. It was six weeks since my first chemo. And so far, absolutely nothing has happened. No hair fall-out. No de-swelling. Nothing. So I'll just wait then, shall I? I can't face today. Hey, future, it seems we might not get to meet after all.

Today is chemo day. I haul myself out of bed, into some ill-fitting clothes and eventually make it to the Royal Marsden in one piece. Sweating profusely like someone with cancer, but pretty much in one piece. The first nurse I see doesn't quite manage to conceal her 'oh fuck, he looks like shit' look. She sends me down for my 'bloods' straight away. The same woman always takes my blood. She never smiles. She always sighs. Loud and long sighs. She taps and prods and anaesthetises and pricks and pulls and labels with steely cold efficiency. I am used to it by now. I quite like it in a perverse kind of way. This is no time for needle phobia. If you have been given a cancer diagnosis, a few pricks are the least of your worries (stop it!).

Today is chemo day. I am sitting in the waiting room. I am waiting (that's what you do in waiting rooms) to see the consultant before embarking on my third course of chemo. This cancer thing can too often feel inexorably lonely. Like you're crawling through the Sahara on your hands and knees with no water and nobody around for miles and miles except a tiny screen in the corner of the sky that is showing you how beautiful and cool and charmed everybody else's life appears to be. Everything seems to be taking a slow-motion amount of time today. My skin throbs and sweats. My head spins. My world's in a blur. I try to read something to pass the time but whenever I try focusing on an individual word, that word leaps off the page and pulsates

pulsates

pulsates

pulsates

and buzzes

buzzzzzzzes

around the room, taunting me and goading me to catch it and nail it down. I don't have the focus or the desire even to begin to try to return it to its rightful place. The best I can do is just look at the peculiar glossy pictures of the obligatory hospital **Hello***-type magazines. Or* **OK!** *Er, right now, NO.*

Seconds and minutes hang around as if they are going out of fashion.

Today is chemo day. Eventually, the junior oncology blah blah comes and sits down next to me and as gently as she possibly can tells me that the reason I feel fucked is because I am fucked and the chemo routine I have been having is just not working and the dark shadow between my lungs has decided to grow rather than shrink and they need to attend to this right now and the only way they can do that is by admitting me right now in order to work out how to reverse the situation and there isn't a minute to waste and my immune system is in serious danger of shutting down completely and if that happens then it could be very serious very serious indeed and there really is no time to waste and would I like to call someone to fetch some things for me and if I just wait here she will get a porter and a nurse to take me to a ward and she or one of her colleagues will be down to see me in the ward later and not to worry because this is what happens at the beginning of chemo to some degree it's trial and error and they need to learn what works and what doesn't work with this particular case and they can only do that by monitoring me and the situation and that I am likely to be in hospital for no more than ten days and by then they will be sure to have found a cocktail more suited to my needs and I will just go and find that nurse to look after you.

Now, to be fair, she *did* talk slightly more slowly than that. She did take one or two breaths. She *was* looking me in the eye when she was telling me this. She *was* really gentle and seemingly caring. She delivered the news as if it was fresh just for me rather than just something she had delivered to countless patients that week. I was nodding like an ever-nodding thing and doing a bad impression of someone who was taking all of this in.

CREEP

It began to creep up on me during the bit where she was talking about my immune system. It slowly filled me up and filled me up till I was fit to completely fracture. And the straw that finally broke cancer boy's back wasn't the fucked immune system or the growing mass inside me or the serious danger.

It was the ten days.

- Ten days of hospital.
- Ten days of incarceration.

- Ten days of being reminded of the reality of this right-now situation.
- Ten days of not taking the first show I was ever going to direct to the Edinburgh Festival. And that is the one thing that I absolutely knew had to happen. For my sanity. For my soul. Saying no to Edinburgh would have been like my future slamming the door in my swollen face. An acceptance that *this* is my future now. And, believe me, I was not ready for *this*.

I am desperately treading water trying to keep afloat. I might sink. I might swim. I don't have control over all the circumstances that might pull me under. I am not brave. I am not battling. I am just doing 'now'. 'Battling cancer' implies a lever of proactivity that I don't feel I have. It implies that I am literally staring cancer down, eyeball to cancerous eyeball, dressed in full and rather fetching armed combat gear, ready to pounce for its jugular when I catch a glimpse of its weak spot. If it has one. If only that were true, that would make things so much simpler.

Today is chemo day. I sit in a corridor in a hospital in South Kensington and shake my head and mumble and shake my head and sob. I am grieving for my now. My present. The oncologist is more than adamant that any course of action other than being admitted would be dangerous for my health. I am not an oncologist but I know that isn't true. Through my crazed hysteria I have the clarity to see that the symbolism of letting go so easily will haunt me for the rest of my illness. And that won't be helpful or healthy. I know I have to fight this. Just this once. I know that I am right. I know that going to Edinburgh is much healthier right now than staying in hospital.

I know I am right. Know I am right. Know I am. Won't budge. Won't budge. Won't budge. Won't. Can't.

Today is chemo day. It takes a while, but there comes a point when the nurse and the oncologist look at each other and agree to my demands. They know what has to be done. They go into situation management mode.

> *a) Accommodate his need to get to Edinburgh.*
> *b) Make sure he doesn't die along the way.*

And the doctors' and nurses' flexibility and understanding just underlines my newly discovered understanding that the National Health Service is an incredible institution. I was given the option to be treated privately at the beginning of this saga but my instinct told me I would feel safe in the hands of the NHS. And I do.

Today is chemo day. One of the upsides to spending so much time in hospital is to be able to watch the human machinations of the place in action. I have become fascinated by its natural ebb and flow, its routines, and, most of all, by the working relationships of the doctors and nurses and especially how defined they are in their roles. It is like watching a 3D version of ER. *As a general rule the nurses are more empathetic and doctors/consultants are slightly more aloof but that doesn't feel wrong. It feels like the optimum way to maximise their skills. It also means that often, when they are working together, a magical synergy occurs that can produce extraordinary and surprising results. Such is the case here. It feels incredibly moving to watch the nurses and doctors kick into action around me. It makes me feel important and unique and cared for and, most of all, it makes me feel listened to. And that is the single most essential medicine at this point. The reality is that they are just doing their job and being fucking brilliant at it. And young George Clooney is in charge, of course. No, scrap that. They are all Clooney as far as I am concerned.*

Today is chemo day. There is definitely a debilitating disease called second-opinion-itis. I understand that people want to be sure, want the confidence of more than one diagnosis, but where does it, end? Whose opinion DO you end up trusting? For me, I just want to get on with it, and second and third opinions take an awful lot of time.

INSTINCT

My whole life has been based on instinct. The biggest lesson is to have the confidence to trust that instinct most of the time. And that's not easy. With my diagnosis and pretty much all my treatment, I couldn't find a rationale to doubt what was being said to me. I put myself and my life in the hands of professionals, and I had no reason to think I knew better than them. Medically speaking anyway. And in moments like this, for instance, when I **needed** to be heard, that mutual trust that we had built up allowed a dialogue and a creative solution to be found to a rather tricky, delicate and difficult problem.

And the word 'grace' was invented for moments like this. Moments where everything fell into alignment. Everyone working together at the same tempo and at the maximum of their abilities to produce an outcome that was best for everybody. It was a bit like the most creative moments in a technical rehearsal in the theatre. A kind of quiet and profoundly proactive hum permeates the air. The calm is interspersed with moments of mania. Good mania. Rewarding mania. Creative mania.

Today is chemo day. The medical staff have a plan. And we all sit round a table like adults and talk through the plan. I say 'like adults' because through most of this illness I have felt like a five-year-old, an eight-year-old and a fourteen-year-old respectively:

- *The five-year-old doesn't understand enough to know more than something hurts and he needs to cry about it.*
- *The eight-year-old knows too much. He sort of understands. He knows things are bad but is too shy to ask the scary grown-ups for stuff that might make him feel better.*
- *The fourteen-year-old is trying desperately to be grown up about it all. He is working very hard to hide his pain and his fear.*

Today, because of the generosity and spirit of the doctors and nurses, I am a young adult taking everything in and trying to work out what my opinions on all this stuff might be. It's both daunting and strangely calming all at once. Daunting because you are being given a little bit of control of your life back and you'd better not fuck it up, but calming because you have been given a little bit of control of your life back and you'd better not fuck it up.

THE PLAN

The plan is quite simple. If I allow them to admit me now, they will give me intensive treatment over the next two days. They will then discharge me. I will fly up to Edinburgh for three days armed with a case full of drugs. In four days' time, I will return to London and be admitted again for further intensive treatment. What occurs after that can be discussed at a later date.

Today is chemo day. My heart almost explodes with admiration and thanks for the amazing way they have dealt with difficult young me. The adrenaline that I am feeling at this instant is a perfect cover for any fear that might be lingering around inside. I have a focus and a purpose for the next seven days and that's just awesome. I immediately kick into action, changing flights, accommodation etc. A smog of tunnelled activity surrounds me. I am allowed home for an hour to get some stuff, talk to some people and return. I don't even have to resort to crying to get my own side room. The nurses are on my team. We are all in this one-off, feature-length episode together.

Yesterday was chemo day. And Debbie comes to visit and she brings stuff. I always like it when close friends come to visit because the stuff they bring is normally good stuff. Debbie wrote the play that I am directing in Edinburgh. She is also in it. She is also a uniquely caring, empathetic and understanding woman as well as being a lover of the finely crafted joke. As you may have gathered by now, so am I. She is the ideal visitor for this moment. We are on the same Edinburgh team so it feels like she understands. She is a close friend who has been there from the beginning so I never feel the need or the pressure to explain anything. More importantly, in the moments where the harsh reality of the now starts to rear its ugly head, she has a unique ability to find the right bad gag for the right bad situation. Which never fails to cheer me up. Can I make it up to Edinburgh? Yes you Can-Sir.

I spend two hard-core days in hospital with every possible drug being pumped inside me. The doctors are trying to arrest my decline at the same time as attempting to make a decision about the best course of treatment from now on.

THROUGH THE CANCER GLASS

At times like this, despite putting all my faith and trust in the hands of the Marsden medical team, I would get lost in the vortex of the cancer looking-glass. The huge world above me was spinning. I could no longer distinguish people's voices. It was just constant white-coat medical-related chatter. However, every decision was being relayed to me and a plan for my temporary release was being drawn up. And, despite feeling like a tiny gravity-free molecular speck in a gigantic world, I was invigorated, liberated and empowered.

Three days ago was chemo day. In the blink of a crusty eye I was on a plane to Edinburgh. I was exhausted and exhilarated. The exhilaration wasn't really excitement for what was to come, it was a bit more complex than that. I think it was to do with the power of knowing I had wrested back a bit of control. I had stared into the abyss that life was offering me, stood up to it and refused to budge. I was not laughing in its face because there wasn't a great deal of laughter going on but I sure as hell was not backing down. In the cancer 'who blinks first' competition, I was not blinking. And not blinking. And not blinking. And not blinking. My eyes were watering to fuck. The rest of my face was contorted with the extreme effort of it all but there was no way on God's earth that I was going to blink. If I blinked, I may as well have died. If I blinked , it meant I'd surrendered and that was just not an option.

To paraphrase the great Boss himself (Bruce Springsteen. Not God. Though they may be one and the same.), never retreat and definitely never surrender.

Five days ago was chemo day. I was sitting alone at some trendy café just off the Royal Mile. In Edinburgh. My table was swimming with flyers for a thousand shows. People in outlandish costumes were shoving yet more flyers at me and shouting things.

'Not altogether shit,' says the *Scotsman*. 'Two-for-One this afternoon only. And tomorrow maybe, if you want!'

What normally would just annoy the total fuck out of me, now became this strange aching thing of beauty. A symbol of all I was about to be forced to give up. And I breathed it in. Tried to make it last. But it didn't. Last. It wouldn't. It couldn't. And nostalgic sadness enveloped me and started to strangle me. Tomorrow disappeared. I stopped breathing. The world went white noise. I sat there. And I sat there. And I sat there. Paralysed. In a singular moment of ice-cold time. However hard I tried, however hard I scrunched my face up and squeezed my brain, I just couldn't breathe. I couldn't see into the future. I tried. I tried so hard but the future was a blank to me. And I couldn't breathe. I could cry but I couldn't breathe. And I cried. And cried. And cried.

And it wasn't to do with death. It was to do with the unknown. It was to do with the realisation that from this day forward I had nothing ahead of me. Ahead of me there was just a void. A simple hissing void. The world around me seemed minuscule and every second felt like a lifetime. And I sat there forever. And I didn't move. Didn't want to move. Didn't even think I knew how to. But eventually I had to. Move. Eventually.

I had a show to direct! And that's the point. I had to try to find a way to get beyond the paralysis and keep on moving.

And I did. And you have to.

You put one foot in front of another and in small, slightly unsteady footsteps, you move to the next phase in your life. And however treacherous those footsteps might be, you do have to keep going. Got no choice. And that's what bravery is. Keeping on going, however many obstacles life tries to put in your way. However paralysing life might try to make you feel. And you get five stars in the *Scotsman* for that.

SEX AND CANCER, PART TWO
– THE CANCER SWAGGER

Like in all these cancer tales, contradictions abound. Sex may have been my *lingua franca* but cancer seemed to have changed all the rules that I was previously so well versed in.

One of the side effects of chemotherapy isn't horniness. Not one of the most common ones, anyway.

Coupled with that, you aren't necessarily looking your best:

- You (me) may have no hair.
- You (me) may be puffed up to the nines by the steroids.
- You (me) may have strawberry bloodshot eyes from drugs and lack of sleep.
- You (me) may have 350 mouth ulcers.

The steroids and the mouth ulcers and the no hair and the no sleep are bad enough, but I've saved the worst side effect till last:

The No Arse.

I kid you not.

As if life couldn't get any worse, my oldest and most brutally honest friend Tort pointed out that my most prized asset, the one thing I had in common with The Boss, the one part of my anatomy that is fail fucking safe, had gone. Gone. Stolen from me. By a chemical arse thief. By a drug-pushing bottom burglar. Wait. I think a bottom burglar is something different. Anyway. One careful owner. Not much mileage on the clock etc. That's the true tragedy here.

And the most frustrating thing of all?

I didn't need to know! I could have spent my whole time oblivious to it.

I can't see my arse. It's behind me. *Was* behind me. Now it's been replaced by a flat, cheekless, plumpless mass of nothingness.

AND I DIDNT NEED TO FUCKING KNOW.

So all in all, **not** particularly looking or feeling my best, I might just have to stick to fantasy.

That thought didn't make me depressed, it just made me a bit sad, because I knew that skin on skin right now would be revitalising. And that's what I needed more than anything. **Rejuvenation**.

And somehow, despite feeling desperately unsexy, I managed to find it. There are many reasons why you might want sex when you have cancer:

- To get out of your thinking head and immerse yourself in the world of the physical. In other words, **doing rather than being** and discovering a brief physical escape axis.
- To trick yourself into thinking that you just might be normal. In that moment. You might be *able* to do the things and, more poignantly, *want* to do the things you could do before you were ill.
- To find a release – a chemical release – that might be impossible to find any other way. Without being over-graphic about it, that release surely must be good for you. When I say you, I mean me. And even if, for a brief moment (what's new!), that release is beauty and normality and freedom.

I didn't feel sexy but I certainly did have a bit of that cancer swagger. I think the thing that makes the cancer swagger attractive is that it is completely without pretension and effort.

It just IS. There really was nothing more to lose. I had lost almost everything else up to that point.

What did I really care if someone didn't find me attractive?

Having said I didn't care, that can't be entirely true as I *did* often make more than a little bit of an effort to make myself look slightly less alien-like. The fifteen steroids I was taking a day would make my already large head puff up to an almost comical degree. I got to know that if I stopped taking them, it would be about four days before my head went back to 'normal'. Those steroids were a big part of preventing my immune system from collapsing. But if I had a 'date' on a Saturday, I would stop taking the steroids on the Monday before.

Why would I put myself at risk for a flirtation or a brief meaningless sexual interlude? Well, why wouldn't I? Everybody was looking after my body. Nobody was attending to my soul. I was just paying it some much needed attention with little mutual acts of love. Spurts of love. Sexual love maybe. But love all the same. And that was my language. And it didn't require words. Before, during or after.

The language of sex is so expressive that the spoken word is often superfluous. No explaining, no theorising, no investigating. Just sex.

Don't get me wrong: I am the number one proponent of the highly vivid and often graphic use of words during sex. Nothing better. But sometimes silence is bewitching. The sound of breath, bed springs and gentle bodily collisions can be achingly wonderful. And in the cancer context, where the right words are not always easy to find, that shared passionate sexual silence can be heart-stopping. Sometimes almost is!

It is somebody's way of showing me that they care, that they are with me, that I am not alone. And because they think you might break, they are often careful to be as tender and gentle as they possibly can be. And that's alluring and moving, too.

Having said that, sometimes you want it hard. Real hard. Hard enough to allow you to forget. To forget and be transported to a pre-cancer, less fragile time. And that hardness is beauty, too. Real escape passionate rough beauty. Normally, though, if you want it hard, you have to initiate it. You have to let them know that you'll be OK. That you won't break.

When I use the word 'they' in this context, it sounds pejorative, casual and disrespectful.

It's not.

I use the word 'they' because:

- **'They'** helped me save myself.
- **'They'** helped my heart sing in times when it was caked in shit.
- **'They'** showed me love in a language I understood more than any other.
- **'They'** showed me passion, compassion and tenderness when I needed it but couldn't ask for it.
- **'They'** helped take away the fear, the pain, the loneliness.
- **'They'** made me feel sexy again.
- **'They'** made me feel normal again.
- **'They'** know who they are.

I'm sure some of '**they**' were also morbidly fascinated to fuck someone who might be on the brink of death.

I would be.

And being on the brink of death leads to a multitude of discoveries. Sex turned from being a physical act that I was pretty *au fait* and comfortable with to a way of communicating things in my heart that I found difficult to express overtly in any other form. And the nuances of that expression became an addiction in itself. This touch means this. This movement means that. It became passionate, heartfelt, tender and irresistible. And

I discovered that it doesn't correlate that tenderness means love and the opposite of tenderness means sex. Oh no! It's much more complex than that. And if it all sounds so calculating and unromantic, back off. I can do 'instinct'. I can do 'in the moment'. I'm in the theatre, for fuck's sake!

Physical expressions of love were one of the many revelations during my cancer journey that shaped my future. One of the many things I am grateful for. One of the many reasons that I wouldn't change the past.

1995 to 1996.

An unexpected cancer journey laced with an abundance of sex.

Sex with cancer.

Cancer with sex.

ORAL ARMAGEDDON

Imagine one mouth ulcer.

Imagine two.

Four.

Eight.

Sixteen.

Thirty-two.

Shall I go on?

Yes, I shall.

Imagine 64 mouth ulcers.

Imagine 128 ulcers of the mouth (mouth ulcers).

Imagine 256 oral ulcers (mouth ulcers).

Imagine 300 mucosal ulcers (mouth ulcers).

Imagine 347 aphthous ulcers (mouth ulcers).

Imagine 350 canker sores (mouth ulcers).

Imagine 350 mouth ulcers (mouth ulcers).

That's **Three Hundred and Fifty**.

Three hundred mouth ulcers. And fifty more.

At one time. In one mouth. At one time. In one mouth.

If you are wincing as you are imagining this, imagine how I felt. And imagine this. This isn't literary embellishment. It's true. At the heart of my chemo, the side effects were having a ball, going to town, having a field day. I woke up one day with 350 mouth ulcers. Count them.

3

  5

   0.

And I did.

Count them.

Well, that's actually a lie. The two consultants, four doctors and two nurses that were crowded round my bed studying me like I was the headline exhibit in the Circus of Horrors, counted them.

PAINstakingly. Counted them.

They had never seen the like. Apparently.

I am lying in bed in the Marsden. Decisions are being made about me. I am being referred to, but not spoken to. I can actually speak. I can. It hurts like fuck when I do, but I definitely can. I'd like to. Speak. Have a say. In all this. Think they know that? They must know that? Do they know that? Apparently this is unique. Apparently. A unique side effect. Woo-hoo! I have a constant flow of people coming to look and take endless pics. Now and then someone notices that there is a me beyond the insides of my mouth. They smile sweetly with that look of pity a vet must give a dog just before they put him down. I am twenty-eight. I am not eight. I feel eight. Most of the time I feel eight. I am an eight-year-old in that Munch painting. My life right now is one long inner silent scream. Nobody can see that. Luckily. Cos it's not pretty!

They didn't just count them; they took pictures of them 'n' all. From every angle. And they did lots of prodding and lots of poking. Standard doctors and nurses procedure. Prodding and poking! At certain points I think they forgot I was a living, breathing thing. To them, I was just a head (a huge head at that). More specifically, I was just a mouth. I believe they used the five-line counting method thingy so they didn't lose track. Tally marks, I think they're called. It's a quick way of keeping track of numbers in groups of five. One vertical is made for each of the first four numbers. The fifth number is represented by a diagonal line across the previous four. Like so:

卌

Then you count the bundles. There were millions of bundles. This many bundles:

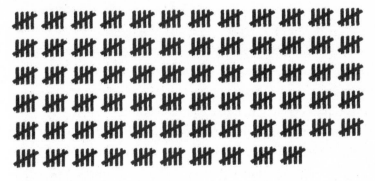

Apparently, the rare extremity of this particular mouth ulcer side effect was due to the specific cocktail of drugs that they were giving me. It appeared that one drug in particular was the main cause of this oral invasion – **Vincristine**. A name like an eighties Italian porn star with the destruction capabilities of a nuclear bomb. A drug used predominantly for blood cancers such as lymphoma or leukaemia. It's the only drug I took any real notice of. I realised very quickly that it wasn't a drug that liked a fair fight. It was a clear liquid, and that in itself can lull you into a false sense of security. It would sooner stab me in the back than face me head-on. So I did some research into Mr V. Cristine. *Encyclopaedia Britannica* rocks!

VINCRISTINE

Cancers form when some cells within the body multiply uncontrollably and abnormally. These cells spread, destroying nearby tissues. Vincristine belongs to the group of drugs called vinca alkaloids. These are often called plant alkaloids because the first of these drugs was developed from the periwinkle plant (vinca). Vincristine works by preventing the cancer cells from entering the dividing stage (mitosis) of their life cycle. This stops the cells from multiplying. Unfortunately,

Vincristine is not able to discriminate between good cells and cancer cells, so it can affect many parts of your body besides the cancer. Since non-cancer cells are better than the cancer cells at repairing the damage caused by Vincristine, the cancer cells die and your normal cells repair the damage so they can resume their normal function. The side effects you experience from Vincristine are a result of this damage to your healthy cells before they have a chance to repair themselves.

And here's the infamous contradiction.

You want to be given the most powerful drugs possible to fight this evil disease. Of course you do. But the more powerful they are then probably the more insidious the side effects are.

So it's lose lose, even when you win.

While we are on the subject, some of the syringes that the nurses used for the chemo were absolutely humungous. And they often contained flamboyantly colourful liquids. I dreaded the moment I saw the nurse heading my way with comedy-sized syringes at the ready. I was trapped in a grotesque cartoon. The nurse sat beside me. Two huge syringes in her hand. One red, one blue.

'*Shall we do it?*' she would say.

I wanted so much to hate her. I wanted so much to turn her into Nurse Ratched from *One Flew Over the Cuckoo's Nest* but she was so sweet and kind and caring that, try as I might, I just couldn't. Dammit! How can someone so lovely and so caring be so comfortable carrying such enormous instruments of evil? And she talked so gently and softly as she administered the poison.

ONE NURSE CHATTING IN THE DARKNESS

This particular nurse liked to chat to me about life, love and the world. Maybe she thought, as I was younger than her average patient and just a little bit cheeky, that it would be fun to engage in general small talk. Or maybe this was her usual distraction method. Either way, she chatted non-stop.

'*Ooo, chat, chat, chat, the world, the world, bits of gossip, chat, chat, chat, the odd flirt, ooo, chat chat, chat.*'

At first I would respond.

'*Ooo, reply, reply, reply, oh yes the world, the world, strange flirting reciprocation, ooo, reply, reply, reply.*'

I was going through the talking motions but the whole time I had my eyes glued to the oversized syringes. I was pondering how ridiculously slowly that red liquid was entering my veins. After a few weeks of treatment, the flow of the liquids became a nightmare and the sweet sound of the nurse's voice sounded like the grating of a hundred fingers on a hundred blackboards.

What I wanted to say to the nurse was:

'*Please. Please. Please. Stop this constant, inane, brain-aching chatter. It's not helping. Not. NOT. NOT. Please, please, please just give this cancer boy a bit of fucking peace. Is that too much to ask?*'

What I actually said was nothing.

Well, when I say 'nothing', what I mean is that I developed this tactic of fake sleeping. I would spend the first couple of minutes '*reply, reply, reply*' and as I watched the beginnings of the liquid pumping into me, I would do some really bad '*I'm drifting off to sleep*' acting. I had to be careful that it didn't get confused with just resting my eyes as that would leave the door open for more nurse '*chat, chat, chat*'. So I had to put in a few fake comedy snores here and there.

I was in a cartoon after all.

Obviously I wasn't just escaping from the sound of the nurse's voice. Even I am not stupid enough to think that. I surprised myself by not being able to just shrug off chemo as a thing that had to be done. It became an immense psychological obstacle. The syringes and the chemicals became symbols of the uncontrollable cells running amok inside me. The whole routine became the enemy. I think the fact that I couldn't load the gun and fire the bullets myself but had to rely on someone else was just another way that this cancer thing made me feel like a child again.

It was all out of my control. All way out of my comfort zone and in a place where I was unable to use my charm or even my perverse humour to escape from the grim reality that was now.

When the darkness comes (and however much you might think that you are different, the darkness **will** come), don't fight it off too hard. You need to allow a space for it. A space big enough for you to feel it but not so big that you can't control it. If you allow it to envelop you too much, the effort of shaking it off will be immense. And, believe me, you're going to need all the strength you've got in the months to come. But if you dismiss it too lightly it will turn up and torture you when you least expect it. And torture is normally not fun. Normally.

Cancer was the drill sergeant major, pinning me down. Its spittle in my face:

'WHAT? YOU THINK THIS IS A GAME? YOU THINK THIS IS ANOTHER OF THOSE SITUATIONS THAT YOU CAN JUST CHARM YOUR WAY OUT OF? NO. THAT SELF-DEPRECATING CHARM SHIT DON'T WORK ON ME. NO, NO. THIS IS REAL, MOTHERFUCKER. THIS IS REAL FUCKING LIFE. YOU HAVE CANCER, MOTHERFUCKER. THIS AIN'T NO GAME. YOU CAN'T FLIRT OR JOKE YOUR WAY OUT OF THIS ONE, BOY. BECAUSE THAT'S ALL YOU ARE. A BOY. JUST A BOY. THIS IS REAL-FUCKING-LIFE RIGHT HERE. OR DEATH. THIS IS NOW. RIGHT NOW. GET USED TO IT. BOY! LIFE OR DEATH. YOU DECIDE!'

And when cancer gets noisy, sometimes the only thing to do is just close your eyes, put your hands over your ears and go:

'BLAH, BLAH, BLAH, BLAH, BLAH, BLAH, BLAH, BLAH, BLAH.'

Don't knock that tactic. It's a good one. Sometimes it's the only way.

Escape is escape is escape is amazing. **Escape** feels like you have been handed this uber-tricky situation solely to challenge yourself into switching on the engine of your under-used imagination! And that's the genius of your mind. Of your dreams. You can escape *to* anywhere. Escape *from* anything. For a moment or two. Or even three. If you're lucky.

On the flip side, curiously, sometimes embracing the harsh reality of the situation, facing it head-on, can be weirdly liberating, too.

For instance, if you have 350 mouth ulcers and you can't speak and you can't eat and it is a military operation to take even one teaspoon of lukewarm 'Not-even-Heinz' tomato soup – sip of water, weenie bit of soup, washed down by a tiny drop of water, soup, water, soup, water, soup etc., adding up to one teaspoon of soup every ten minutes while your mother sits next to you trying to hide the fact that this is breaking her heart – what would be the oddest or most perverse thing you could do?

Anybody?

Well, with 350 mouth ulcers, the most perverse thing you could do might be to take a large salt and vinegar crisp between your fingers. To open your oral cavity that has the 350 mouth ulcers in it. To slowly deposit the salt and vinegar crisp in your mouth-ulcer-ridden orifice – being very careful not to break it. The crisp, that is, not the mouth. To rest the salt and vinegar crisp on your tongue and then slowly bring your tongue up so that the crisp connects to the roof of your mouth!

Why would you want to do that? Why? WHY?

Well, good question.

My only answer would be the same as people give to the perennial question, 'Why climb Mount Everest?'

Cos it's there!

I will never have this opportunity again (I hope), and so in the spirit of wanting to embrace the uniqueness of this cancer journey it is something I just had to do. Plus, in truth, I was aware that it might make a good story for any book I may think about writing in twenty years' time.

It also taps into the heart of what I am trying to say.

This was a special time. It might not be especially wonderful. A lot of the time it was specially fucking awful. But it *was* special:

- The more I embraced it.
- The more I tried to take something new from every difficult moment.
- The more I forced myself to escape from the darkness by exploring new coping strategies.
- The more I used this opportunity to do things and try things that I would never imagine I could do.

The more I would surprise myself by how much inner strength I had and by how possible it became to enjoy rather than endure the now.

And, twenty years on, I am grateful to the me that I was back then for pushing myself not to take it lying down. Literally. So many of those decisions inform who I am now and the choices I make every day. Either consciously or, more interestingly, subconsciously. Any insight I may have now comes from the twenty-eight-year-old me not sleepwalking through it all. It comes from him being curious about experiencing each moment to the full, no matter how crazy that might feel to others at the time. Hence the crisp thing.

Having said that, my pathological hatred of the act of having big, multi-coloured chemicals injected into me seemed to be quite contradictory to the idea of me being open to all new experiences on this journey. I wanted to go through this illness with my eyes wide open but I wanted to go through the biggest chemical procedure within this illness with my eyes wide shut.

And to this day I don't really know quite why that is. It is something to do with the psychological and the emotional being too close to the surface. They felt like they would suffocate me with their all-pervasiveness. They throbbed my head with too much 'stuff'. Those too overpowering fuckers, Mr Psychological and Mr Emotional, sat like ticking bombs on my forehead and deliberately pressed down and down and down. Hard. They wanted me to know they were there. Wanted me not to forget why I was there. They pushed so hard that everything was a blur. I couldn't escape them. And I think that was the point.

This was a weekly moment where I couldn't use my Raz tools to set myself free. And that made me feel bereft because my toolbox has always been my escape route. My toolbox has always been equipped with weird shit that could get me out of most scrapes.

In the **Raz Toolbox,** there are a number of fail-safe tools. These include:

THE FLIRTATION TOOL

The flirtation tool guarantees that you can soften most situations with a smile, a touch, a sparkle or just a wee bit of sexual frisson (rather than a sexual frisson bit of wee; that's completely different). Raz likes to think the flirtation tool works well with most people but it is especially successful with older women and gay men. The flirtation tool can also be utilised with straight men. You just have to wrap it up in a somewhat less sparkly form.

THE INAPPROPRIATE TOOL

The inappropriate tool is more useful than anyone will ever imagine. It is pure escape. It is a major weapon of mass distraction. It is deflection. It's used like this: you're in a situation where you or someone around you is feeling awkward. For whatever reason. You explode open the inappropriate tool, and people are so busy commenting and outraging about your wilful act of inappropriateness that they forget the utter awkwardness that just preceded it. Simple.

THE DAD-JOKE TOOL

Don't ever underestimate the power and usefulness of the dad-joke tool. It's yet another deflection tool. It can be used in most situations but it's most helpful when needing to bring an unwanted conversation to an abrupt end. Imagine the scenario. You are having dinner in a Greek restaurant and the dinner bore is boring the arses off the other guests. (By the way, the old adage DOES apply here: if there's five of you at a dinner table and you see no dinner bore, guess what that makes you?) And the dinner bore doesn't stop. He goes on and on and on. And even the waiter coming up barely stops him. So you put the dad-joke tool into operation.

The Greek waiter says: *'Can I take your order?'*

And you say: *'Can you recommend something? This menu's all Greek to me!'*

Now I can honestly say that particular joke is so bad, even *I* wouldn't use it. But I needed to visit extremity to make my point. *My* dad jokes are much wittier and more erudite. The point is that a really bad dad joke can hang around long after the groans. So if you are really smart, you will use that moment to deflect the attention away from the dinner bore onto something or someone more interesting. Like yourself for instance!

Like I said, for me these tools are fail-safe. They have been my protection and preservation for all the years I care to remember. But for some reason, in the maelstrom of chemo, my toolbox and everything else I had to protect myself with was ripped from me. I was naked and disarmed. A defenceless child.

And nothing helped. No distraction techniques, no tools, nothing. In the purity of those endless chemo minutes, there was no escape. And those minutes *were* endless. Nothing could speed them up. I was swimming in slow motion, underwater, against the tide. And it seemed like it would never end. *Make it end. Make it end. Make it end. Make it end.*

The longest journey on the longest day into the longest night.

The rest of the time I was quite good at finding distraction opportunities, but on chemo day Mr Psychological and Mr Emotional were boss. They would command you not to forget. They would command you to have at least one hour a week where you were awake to the situation you were in. Bastards. On that day at that time, you had zero power, strength or wilful desire to fight them.

Oh, and how *does* a salt and vinegar crisp feel in a mouth full of 350 ulcers?

DUH! It feels like the most painful fucking thing you have ever felt in your whole life.

It feels like 350 daggers jabbed into your mouth at once.

It feels like Oral Armageddon.

I'M A SECRET POSITIVE THINKER

I'm a secret positive thinker. I am. At least I think I am. I'm fairly positive I am. Or am I a secret *wannabe* positive thinker? I would love to be a truly positive person. On the rare occasion that I've met one, I've always envied them. I did when I was ill and I do now.

When I was ill I hid my positivity jealousy under a veil of cynicism. And only at night, alone, under my covers, would I unveil myself and will myself to be positive. I tried really hard. I really did. But it was just too abstract a concept for my singular brain. I would lie there in the middle of the night, close my eyes, scrunch my whole face up tight and desperately try to bewitch my way to positivity land.

Positive thoughts.

Come on, Raz.

Positive thoughts.

Come on, Raz.

Come on.

I hear a deep growl coming from the heart of my soul. Aaaaaaaa aaaaaaaaaaaaaaaaaaaaaaaaaaaaaaaaaaaaaaaaaaaaaaaaaaaaaaaaaaaaa aaaaaaaaaaaaaaaaaaaaaaaaaaaaaaaaaaaaaaaaaaaaaaaaaaaaaaaaaaaaa aaaaaaaaaaaaaaaaaaaaaaaaaaaaaaaaaaaaaaaaaaaaaaaaaaaaaaaaaaaaa aaaaaaaaaaaaaaaaaaaaaaaaaaaaaaaaaaaaaaaaaaaaaaaaaaaaaaaaaaaaa aaaaaaaaaaaaaaaaaaaaaaaaaa.

POSITIVITY.

You can do it. Come on.

Come the fuck on!

Wait a moment. Just one moment. Before I do this, what is this? What is it? What exactly is a positive thought? It really does seem so abstract to me. More of a concept than an actual active thing. What actually is it? Hmm?

?

?

Never mind, let's do this.

*Let's do **positivity**.*

OK. OK. OK.

C'mon, Raz. Try again. C'mon!

OK. OK. I am squeezing my eyes tight shut. Squeezing. Squeezing. Squeezing. My fingers are clenched. My bottom is clenched. Every single little bit of me is clenched.

Squeeze.

Squeeze.

Come on. It's almost there. I know it. I can feel a tiny positive thought about to poop out. I mean pop out.

Yes? Yes? YES?

Nope!

Sometimes, when I was under those covers trying to force a bit of positivity out I made myself laugh at how ridiculous that actually was. How maddening. How odd. How funny. And I immediately found a semblance of serenity in that thought.

But the act of trying to feel positive and not exactly succeeding often feels worse and more painful than not trying at all. I am grateful for my cynical bones as they kept my mind from flying off in any direction, high or low. They allowed me to at least try to exist in that moment. They allowed me to at least try to see life as it really was and respond to it accordingly. And that's quite a healthy way to exist when you're not healthy and you're worried about not existing.

Rather than trying to be positive in the abstract , it's much more about **not** being negative.

Not Being Negative is much more positive than any **P**ositive **M**ental **A**ttitude mantra!

Not Being Negative is very day-to-day doable. Everyone can do it. Anyone can do it.

On a day-to-day basis, we are **Not Being Negative** loads of times, hundreds of times even.

The reason that **Not Being Negative** really worked for me is because it released me to forget yesterday and not to worry about tomorrow. It released me to take today and try to just live it. Maybe that's just positivity wrapped up in another form, but there's much less disappointment in looking at things that way.

Positivity feels intangible. And because it feels so intangible and abstract and out of reach, I was left with that nagging, sinking, empty feeling inside that I was somehow letting the cancer club down and, more importantly, I was letting myself down. And that definitely wasn't healthy. Age has taught me how to embrace the moments in life, however fleeting, where positivity feels real and active and right. And that's the point. True positivity has to go hand in hand with sometimes harsh reality; otherwise it's just vapid froth and air.

People always asked me if I thought I was going to die. Did I think about death? Yes, of course I did. It's in the cancer diagnosis contract. Did I think I was going to die? Well, no, I didn't. I thought about how people might react if I did die (I love a drama), but I didn't actually think I would. Die. And that's absolutely about me living my life in a 'not negative' way. And that really worked for me.

CONFIDENCE

A close relative of positivity is confidence. *Confidence* can be both how you feel inside and how you present yourself to the world. They are not mutually exclusive. Indeed, sometimes one fuels the other.

You are feeling shit inside and have no confidence. In yourself or your ability to fight this fucker. Sometimes just faking it and presenting to the world an external picture of someone who is bright, breezy, puffed-up (not by steroids but by life) and has a certain swagger can somehow fool *yourself* into believing that you are *actually* feeling those things inside. You forget yourself for a bit and believe your own hype. It can help. It can alleviate things for a while. Even a short while. And that's better than no while. The comedown can be quite major, though. **Fake confidence cold turkey.**

When my brain kicked in and the positivity induced (fake or otherwise) endorphins disappeared, my insides were reminded of my previous pain. But, faking it *is* a coping mechanism and for a while I did believe it. More than that, it felt good. So now the trick was to try to fake it for longer each time. And the longer it got the more real it got, and the more real it got the less I had to fake it, and the more I believed I could deal with the illness.

More than that, some days I sailed through it, feeling smug that I was more than coping. In some perverse way, I was enjoying it. And that enjoyment was a lot to do with feeling proud of myself for finding ways *not* to surrender to the anguish. Not to feel sorry for myself and not to let the negativity win. A whole lot of NOTS to untie.

It's all semantics really. It doesn't matter what we choose to call it. **Being Positive. Not being negative.** Just words. The more I faced up to the reality of my situation, the more I sculpted my environment to help me deal with that reality, the less thought I gave to tomorrow and the more equipped I felt to try to enjoy whatever life chose to throw at me today.

CANCER VERSUS GAMBLING, PART TWO

In the seemingly endless months between June 1995 and April 1996, I was fighting three separate and yet intrinsically entwined battles:

1) ME VERSUS STAGE 4 NON-HODGKIN'S LYMPHOMA

This wasn't really a fair fight.

I was one lone, slightly odd, belligerent, would-be funny north London Jew.

Cancer was thousands of years old. With an army of billions of cells behind it.

It had mounds of experience as to how to break down my brittle defences.

I **had** me, a couple of pamphlets and a few doctors armed with drugs.

In 1995, I didn't even have Google to help me.

I had a sense of humour.

That was my biggest weapon. My cancer would get increasingly frustrated by that sense of humour. Every time it pushed out a side effect, it would sit back and just expect that to be the one that would make my resistance disappear. But it hadn't reckoned on my retaliation missile. My comedy arrow had staggeringly pinpoint accuracy.

Cancer hated that I had a weapon. It began to up the ante.

The mouth ulcer weapon was its attempt to sink my *Belgrano* (that's not a euphemism) and to try to shut me up for good. It very nearly succeeded, but it didn't bank on my perversity in adversity.

After that, cancer either lost heart or tried a completely different tactic. It was a petulant child who loathed being ignored. Now and again, it would send out suicide bombers with minor explosives to cause a modicum of havoc. But I could deal with that. I had survived the big stuff, so the rest was manageable. Cancer hated that I was coping. It would try to blindside me at any given opportunity. It almost succeeded. Almost.

2) ME VERSUS GAMBLING

This was a fight that had been going on for an awfully long time. Almost ten years since I'd recognised it as a problem. I never really tried to stop it because I never really wanted to. I made proclamations all the time. But nobody believed them – because I never believed them. The truth is that I was head over heels in love. With gambling. It gave me everything I needed: adrenaline, excitement, escape. It wasn't better than sex. It WAS sex. It was sex and love all wrapped into one big gambling maniacal thing. I'm not good with love, but I'm good with sex!

Gambling was one of the few things that I knew how to love. I totally loved gambling. And gambling totally loved me.

We would fight all the time but our make-up sex was off the scale.

Our **love** was unconditional.

Win or lose, I would always **love** gambling.

I would **hate** it too.

Hate it more than I have hated anything or anyone before or since.

But, **love** or **hate,** it made me really *feel* things. That's what I really loved.

And then one day it made me feel numb.

When the numbness takes over, that's when you really have to worry. That's when your intake capacity is so high that only a binge of epic proportions will impinge on the deadness. And you have to go further and further to find that high again.

The vicious circle out of control vortex is set to max.

3) ME VERSUS THE NOTION OF STOPPING GAMBLING DESPITE IT SEEMING TO HELP ME GET THROUGH THIS CANCER MADNESS

That was a hard concept to get my head round. Thankfully it wasn't something I was even conscious of at the time. But it was undeniable that the distraction of my gambling addiction was making the day-to-day of cancer living much easier to deal with. That's not to say that being in the midst of a gambling addiction was a breeze. Far from it. But, for good or for bad, the addiction filled every particle of my waking being. The self-hatred altitude was so high that it almost totally consumed everything else. There wasn't a lot of room for cancer. That said, cancer doesn't like being second best so it wasn't going to give up first place without the mother of all fights!

Gambling addiction was so much simpler before the cancer.

BC, I would wake up and know that there was just one thing devouring my mind. Last night's win/loss and the next bet. That haunted abyss inside me was weeping. It was begging to be filled. This was pre-internet gambling days so 11.02 on the first race at Romford was my first opportunity to fill it.

I am in bed. I am in a white cold sweat of disgust wondering what the fuck I am doing with my life. I tell myself I am going to stop. I tell myself this at the same time as I find myself marching towards the bookies. I am in the bookies. I am in the bookies and I am telling myself that I am not actually going to have a bet today. I am telling myself that even if I do have a bet today, it will be my last. I am telling myself that even if it isn't my last, I am in control of it. I am telling myself that I will just have one. Just one bet and then leave. One bet and get on with my day. One bet and get on with my life. And so I have that one bet. And that dog almost wins. It almost wins. And that rush of almost-winning-adrenaline feels good. It fills the chasm. For now. I tell myself that I will win on the next one. I will win and then I will stop. And I do win. I win. That's fucking great. I win. I have a full wallet and I won. And I can't leave now because maybe, just maybe, I am on a winning streak and today could be the day. It could be the day that wipes out all my debts and takes me back to the top and once I am back at the top I am going to stop and it will feel great because I will stop and I will be debt-free and have nothing to chase because I will be debt-free and I will stop gambling and I will get on with my life. And I will no longer wake up wishing I hadn't. Woken up. I will no longer wake up and wish my life would end. And. And. And today will be that day. Today will be. Will be. Will. Be. That. Day. And. And Today. And the next bet. And after lunch. And I need to fill that hunger. And the next. Bet. And. I walk out of the bookies at 5.17. I have been in there for six hours. I stink of other people's cigarettes and ache of self-hatred.

I may have won, I may have lost. It didn't matter. I was sleepwalking through my life. Single-handedly trying to destroy any chance I might have of a future, a career, a life.

And then I was diagnosed with cancer.

I've already said that cancer saved my life. It really did. It focused my life. It, eventually, gave me perspective. And it gave me something to live for. None of that happened immediately and most of it happened unwittingly and indirectly, but it did happen. It was the most complicated year of my life and I still can't quite make proper sense of it some twenty years later.

Days and nights were spent at the casino, at the hospital or watching the OJ Simpson trial.

Cancer and gambling ran in parallel the whole time. They echoed each other and raced each other and goaded each other and fought each other. I was the cancer piggy in the middle of it all.

It *was* a race.

A race to the finish line.

ADDICTION TAKES NO PRISONERS

Addiction identifies your weaknesses and your vulnerabilities and goes straight at them. It has sniffer-dog capabilities. Once it has found its prey it will latch on like a leach and be impossible to discard.

Addiction is the perfect chameleon. Once it's on you and in you it will manifest itself in so many forms. It will do anything to make you love it. To make you feel like it's part of you. That you can't live without it. That you don't *want* to live without it. It is the perfect ying to your yang. It complements you. It makes you think you have become the person you always wanted to be. It fills up the emptiness inside you that nothing or nobody has ever been able to fill before.

And that's its genius.

When you first meet, it feels so good. So right, so thrilling.

Life is so much better with it in your life. It absorbs itself into you. It becomes part of you. Part of your identity. It invades every single bit of you. Not only can you not live without it but you need more and more of it just to keep you on an everyday equilibrium. The more you have, the dirtier you feel. So you need even more. Even more will definitely take you back to the time when just doing it made you feel invincible.

CHASING NOSTALGIA

And that's what you're doing. You're chasing nostalgia. And chasing nostalgia only ever leads to pain. Because you can never go back. But, addiction equals madness and the madness tells you that you CAN go back. You are the Time Lord. You are insuperable. You **can** go back to better times. You can. And that's what addiction is.

It's a **cult**. It's a **cult**. It's a **cult**. It's a **cult**. It's a **cult**. It's a **cult**.

Once addiction's got you in its cult, it will do anything to make you stay. Or, more precisely, it will do anything for you NOT to leave. And this cult takes no prisoners, and its leaders are fucked and evil and will never let you go. Ever. The harder you fight, the more evil they get. The finish line is a place of such surrender that you don't have any fight left to try to escape from it. So you surrender to it. You glorify in it. You accept the inevitable final tragic darkness of it. They have you by the medicated scruff of your cancer neck and they are forcing you towards life's finishing line. And you need shitloads of energy to fight them. Energy that you just don't have.

CULTISH CANCER

Cancer is also pure enemy. It is just as evil and cultish as a gambling addiction. More so:

1. It overtly makes the first move.
2. It is indiscriminate in its targets.
3. It won't give you any early breathing space.
4. It can mutate at will.
5. It laughs at the lengths people have to go to try to destroy it.
6. It laughs in the face of side effects.
7. It forever ups the stakes and the ante.

8. It is deeply arrogant.
9. It needs to be number one.
10. It hates you having other lovers.
11. It will do anything to win.

Winning for cancer is your **death**. Simple as that.

That is the finishing line. Anything less is just unacceptable.

And so in 1995, as summer began to turn to autumn, Cancer and Gambling Addiction were chest-deep in battle. A battle for my life.

'WE'RE IN THE HAT BUSINESS'

Some people said that, when I was young, I had a bit of a Jew-fro with strawberry-blond tendencies. I am not at all sure that that was true!

In actuality, I never really thought much about the pros and cons of my hair. Or hair in general, really. Until I was diagnosed with cancer. And then, that's all people talked about.

I guess that is the iconic cancer image.

Bald.

Naked-bald if it's a man or bandana-bald if it's a woman.

It was the first picture that came into my head when I realised I had cancer. Not necessarily the first thought but definitely the first picture, and it became my way of telling people about my diagnosis.

'We're in the hat business. We're in the hat business.'

I loved the fact that it took some people a while to cotton on. So much so that I had to explain it to them and then repeat the 'soften the blow' phrase. Which sort of defeated the point.

'We're in the hat business.'

'You what?'

*'We're in the **hat** business.'*

'The what?'

'The h-a-t business.'

'Oh. We are?'

'What?'

'In the hat business?'

'YES!'

'Raz.'

'*YES!*'

'*What the fuck are you talking about?*'

'*OH! Well. It's nothing to worry about. I'm fine. Well, not fine. OK. Well, sort of OK. I mean, I will be fine so don't worry about it. Nothing really to worry about.*'

'*WHAT? WHAT IS NOTHING TO WORRY ABOUT?*'

'*Oh. I have non-Hodgkin's lymphoma.*'

'*Shit.*'

'*Yes.*'

'*Shit.*'

'*It's fine. I'm fine.*'

'*OK.*'

'*OK.*'

'*Erm. Raz? What is it?*'

'*What is what?*'

'*The non-thingy lymph thingy.*'

'*OH. It's. Well, it's a type of cancer. Of the lymph glands.*'

'*Oh shit. I'm sorry.*'

'*It's fine. I'm fine. So you see, we're in the hat business.*'

'*What? OH OH OH. Yes. Hahaha. I see. Oh shit. Oh shit. OH SHIT! I'm sorry.*'

So you see, it doesn't always go to plan.

But 'we' *were* in the hat business. At least that was my perception of the future. Of *my* future. I didn't really have much to go on. I hadn't really properly known anyone with cancer up to that point. I mean, I had known people, but only from afar and certainly not well enough to know the ins and outs and details and things.

ICONIC-BALD

Up until this point, the iconic-bald was about as deep as my cancer knowledge had taken me. Or maybe it was about as deep as I had wanted to take it. Because up until 1995 BC, apart from the more tabloidy stories of a famous person with cancer or a child braving leukaemia, my personal and thus emotional connection with the illness was very limited.

Pathetically limited, in fact.

BEYOND THE BALD

But now, I was beginning to see things beyond the bald.

I don't make light of the bald. The bald is an extraordinarily strong and sometimes frightening symbol that you or I have cancer. And to many it sums up the despair, the pain and the humiliation we feel. It is a vivid external symbol of what is eating away at us.

Bald to a *man* doesn't have to say cancer. It can say cool. It can say hard. It can say gay. It can say all sorts of things that you can embrace and enjoy. The croupiers at my casino just thought *my* bald was my twenty-eight-year-old fashion statement. Bald doesn't have to say cancer to a man.

To a woman it screams cancer. A deafening, hideous, silent scream.

It remains one of the most painful memories of the whole of my cancer experience. To lie in a day bed on a ward and hear a woman behind a screen wrestling in tears with her wig and her dignity is truly heartbreaking. It was clear that all she wanted was to look in the mirror and see herself. If she could see herself, then she could be herself. Even for just a few moments. And no matter how much she fluffed up the wig, she just couldn't see the she she wanted to see. And the pain and panic in her voice was distressing to hear. She just needed a few moments' respite. A few moments of escape breath.

LET THE BALDNESS BEGIN

I was ready for the bald. At least I thought I was. Ready to retire the Jew-fro with ginger tendencies and be cool. A bald, cool Jew with cancer. Cool.

We *were* in the hat business and, to be in the hat business, we must have hats. Why am I using the royal we meaning me? *We* were in the hat business so *we* needed to buy me hats. See. Not as stupid as I was about to look! And the hats, they started to come in. From all over the globe.

LA,
    Sydney,
        Mexico City,
            New York City,
                Hull City.

Some of the hats were cool, some really NOT so cool, but all heartfelt gestures of thought. In order to make the hat thing really play out, I needed one simple thing to happen. I thought it would happen immediately. Thought that I'd have one dose of chemo and va-voom, I'd be hairless. I genuinely had got it into my head that that's what would happen. I even thought that the hair itself would just magically disappear. Vanish into nowhere. I am not entirely sure *where* I thought the hair would go. Maybe it would just be sucked back into my head. I hadn't really thought that far ahead. I just thought it would go. In an instant.

But it doesn't go.
And it doesn't go.
Weeks have passed now and it still doesn't go.
And more weeks have passed and still it doesn't go.
And it does not go.

FRO STILL NO GO

And, very strangely, my hair NOT going started to really get to me. It was like a badge of honour that I really needed to wear to validate me in some way. I felt like a freak. A fraud. I had hats. But I still had hair. I had cancer. But I still had hair. I had had heavy-duty chemo. But I still had hair.

I don't know why I needed the hair to go so much. I think that, if this thing was going to happen, then I needed it to happen to the max. That way I could feel its full force and see what the fuck I was made of. This wasn't conscious thinking, you understand. The conscious me was in an uncontrollable torrent and I was searching for anything I could grab hold of to stop me from going under. Besides, it felt wrong wearing baseball caps with bits of Jew-fro seeping out over the sides. I looked like Krusty the Clown! Even when my chemo moved from being once every three weeks to weekly did the fro no go. The doctors put it down to me having really strong hair. Whatever the fuck that means. I didn't want strong hair. I wanted no hair.

AND THEN IT HAPPENS

I was lying on my hospital bed listening to my mum chatter on about I don't know what – golf or bridge or Andy Murray, who was only eight at this time – and I lifted my head and a huge mound of my hair was left on the pillow. I don't know why it chose that moment to come out. It just did. I felt a wave of something. I don't really know if it was a happy wave or a sad wave. It was just a wave. I think the wave was a recognition that the iconic symbol of cancer was upon me and that there was no escape. If there is an emotion that combines relief and fear, this was it.

Felief. Or Rear.

LET THE MOULTING BEGIN

And, boy, did it moult. Once it started, it didn't stop. I shed hair from every pore. Every orifice. I did the classic thing of shaving all my hair off before it got the chance to disappear itself. Nobody likes a tufty Jew. But I was not prepared for it all going. It *all* going. And I ended up looking like a big old, puffy-eyed, huge-headed, no-arsed, smooth-skinned newborn.

It made me feel and look like an alien. It also made me feel totally conspicuous and totally invisible all at the same time. Invisible because I didn't really feel like me at all. Me had been displaced by an alien boy. God knows if me was ever coming back.

THE BADGE

It was also curiously comforting and distinctive. Being bald was one thing, being utterly hair-free was quite another. Brought a whole new meaning to the term 'smooth'. But smooth I really was. And born again. Not in a religious way, you understand, but in a soft and vulnerable way. Very vulnerable. And very soft. And other. As I've said, I like 'other'. Other took me out of my cocoon into a place of oddness and otherness and wonder. Odd but strangely thrilling.

My badge had finally arrived and I would try to wear it with pride. Some days that was easier said than done. Some days it wasn't a badge of honour. Some days it was a stark symbol that 'other' didn't always mean magical. It often just meant ill. Not only that, this badge was a long time coming so maybe it would be a long time leaving as well.

And those were the days when it felt like my hair loss had stripped me of my protection and left me vulnerable and open to the world. Not sure how a bit of body hair and a Jew-fro could save me from global malevolence, but without it I felt much more exposed.

HAIR – A NON-MUSICAL FABLE IN TWO PARTS
PART 1: HAIR OF THE BACK

My hairy back was a thing I wore with pride. A thing I had selflessly donated to many women along the way when conversations dried up. When lost for words, let them explore the forest that is my back. Loads of conversation starters there. And even that had disappeared. My personal back jungle wiped out in one foul chemo swoop. Or, rather, in one three-month swoop.

But it hadn't taken long for the hairlessness to become part of me. Part of my identity. In no time at all, it had become a shield, a weapon, a comfort blanket, an enemy and a new best friend (new best friends often disappear without a trace after a year or so, especially if you work in the theatre!). It had given me moments of deep sadness alongside moments of wondrous hilarity.

PART 2: *IL EST CHAUVE COMME UNE BOULE DE BILLARD* (HE IS BALD AS A BILLIARD BALL)

I was going to Paris with a couple of friends for a few days. It had been booked for a while and, even though I was feeling pretty shite, I needed to not cancel it in order to try and convince myself that I could be normal. Do normal things. Have a holiday.

The moment we arrived I knew it was a mistake:

Paris is a walking city.

Paris is a smoking city.

Paris at the weekend is an incredibly busy city.

Not only did I not have the energy for it but it seemed to just amplify the illness. It appeared to be taunting me.

Will this thing ever end? Will I actually escape this thing alive?

As the song of my teens might go:

Every step I take, it's watching me.
Every breath I take, seems like a year off my life.
Every move I make, makes me feel eighty fucking years old.

I could irrationally blame the French. They are an easy target. I am not averse to easy targets. But one of the reasons I love Paris is I love the French. Don't get me wrong, I hate them, too. Like New Yorkers, Parisians live up to and play up to their stereotype. Some can be more than a little bit arrogant. Some can be a touch aloof. And some can make you feel really dumb when you attempt French and it's crap, but I think that is all part of their charm. At least they have character. That's more than can be said for the ----------- (insert your own irrational xenophobic target here).

Today it all felt wrong and difficult and tiring and upsetting. And I didn't want to tell my friends because I didn't want to spoil their mini break. That wouldn't be fair at all. Plus, telling them might make my feeling shit a self-perpetuating vicious circle from which there might be no escape. So I kept it to myself. And just tried to go with the flow. It cost me a fortune in coffees as every twelve steps I insisted that we needed to stop for yet more overpriced refuelling.

And the effort of keeping up a cheery façade is hard for me at the best of times. At this very moment, it was almost killing me. And this wasn't the time for a double homicide.

The trouble with the hairless thing is that not only is it a reminder to you that you have a life-threatening illness but it is a reminder to the rest of the world, too, and that marks you out as someone they will either kill with kindness or take two steps to avoid. So the greatest moments are often those moments when people completely forget and treat you as a normal human being.

Paul was in my hotel room having a shower. The room he and his wife were in only had a bath. Actually, I made that last bit up. In truth, I can't remember why he was in my room having a shower. That's not really relevant to this story. I mean, it is relevant. Of course it's relevant. This is a story about a man in a shower. So the location of the shower and the fact that he was actually *having* a shower are both relevant. The underlying reason *why* he was in *my* room having a shower when he had a perfectly decent room to cleanse himself in has slipped my mind. There must be a perfect explanation for it. But I can't recall it. I apologise for that. It was over twenty years ago so it *is* perfectly understandable that the reason Paul was in my shower and not using his own bathroom facilities might have slipped my mind. Maybe he was in my shower in order for me to have a story to tell in two decades' time? I don't know. I can't remember. I wasn't at my brightest at the time, you see. I had cancer, you know. Did I tell you? So. Not quite as on the button as normal. So apologies for my detail deficiencies. I mean, I could just make it all up. That would be easier. But I am running with the facts here. Trying to at least. So...

Paul was in my shower.

I was on my bed.

Paul: *Razzy.*

Raz: *Uhuh.*

Paul: *Do you have any shampoo with you?*

(Long pause)

Raz: *Erm, erm, not really...*

(Long pause)

Paul: *Oh shit, oh shit, oh shit. I forgot. Oh shit, oh shit. Sorry.*

(Long pause)

Paul: *Shit. Shit. Sorry. Shit.*

(Long pause)

Paul: *I guess that means you didn't bring any? Shit.*

And that awkward exchange was the highlight of my Paris trip. For one brief second, I was normal. I was not an alien. Not someone you had to hesitate before you spoke to. I was the same as you. For once, 'other' can bugger off. At that moment, I was just Razzy, Razzle, Raz, Twatface, whatever your preferred semi-affectionate name might happen to be.

I was just that.

And it was wonderful. It was freedom. And the fact that we laughed so hard about it throughout the tricky Paris trip made it all the more special and life-giving.

And that feeling would stick around long after we got home.

That seems to be what living with cancer is all about.

Holding on to lingering feelings. A series of memories that you can escape to when things get dark. And they will get dark. Darker than you can ever imagine. But you are never alone. The mind is an amazing thing.

So be good to it.

Look after it.

Put a hat on it.

EMBRACING THE SWAGGER

Cancer doesn't give you many gifts. It is more of a taker than a giver. It is the Fagin of illnesses. *Take, take, take, my dears.*

But it does give you one thing.

Status.

Status means many things to many people. For me, it's an internal gauge as to how good or bad, big or small you feel in relation to the next person.

It can be a very fleeting, fluctuating thing. Your status can change in a heartbeat. It is both about how you feel and how others or the world at large make you feel. It is often something that needy people try to paint onto themselves to make them feel better about themselves. That normally involves making others feel worse about themselves.

Status is often intangible and indefinable. Although I'm giving it a damn good go right now. It's a frequently used drama school cliché that you can't play the status of a king. The only way an audience can recognise a king on stage – apart from the shitty, bent, silver foil crown on his head – is by how everyone treats him and how everyone reacts when he is present.

Such is the way if you have cancer.

You are kingly. Or queenly. And the crown fits more snugly around your bald head.

People do treat you differently. They don't have the eloquence they might have previously had around you. They don't quite know what to say. They look at you with a mixture of pity and fear. They visibly shrink in your presence. They try to smile but the flickering fear in their eyes coupled with the quiver in the corner of their mouth betrays their desperate panic at trying to find *le mot juste*.

REDUCTIVE

These are often the people who in your former non-cancerous life you found intimidating or looked up to or felt tongue-tied in front of. These are people like your parents' friends or parents of school friends who, even though you are now a grown person, still make you feel like you are seven years old again. Still manage to reduce you to a quivering dry-mouthed, voiceless, two-foot-tall puerile mess.

Now, it was all change. Now I had cancer, the shoe was well and truly on the other foot. Those people who always seemed like giants to me then seemed small and pale and timid now. They looked sweaty and panicked. Like they walked through the door and were actually confronted with an elephant.

Me.

I am the elephant.

I am an elephant.

I SWAGGER

How did that make me feel? Well, so much better, weirdly. I felt bigger and calmer and more in control. The phrase 'he has the hide of an elephant' made perfect sense. I felt ten feet tall. And, yes, I had a sort of swagger. Not sort of. I had a swagger.

Not the full on 'fuck me' swagger. Not in front of the parents! Besides, I've already talked about that. This swagger was less about the hips and more about a gentle understated confidence.

It was about control.

Despite a desperate lack of control over those aliens eating away at my insides, in this situation I felt more in control than ever. At least more in control than those poor pitying people staring at me across the table. This control puffed me up. It was chemo-free medication. With no side effects. Or, at least, very few. I was released from the nightmare of having to force out a smile all the time. That was everyone else's job. It was about not having to expend my much needed energy on making an effort to make myself feel comfortable. In fact, just the opposite, I had a job to do. A job that would enhance that regal swagger.

YOUR MISSION

Your mission now, if you wish to accept it, is to set up the circumstances where people around you feel calm, at ease and good about themselves. They have overcome their embarrassment and bashfulness and are now able to look you squarely in the eye and talk turkey. Turkey cancer. Or not. Whichever is appropriate. It is YOUR job to make that happen. They can't do it alone. Oh no! And when you see their transformation, it is indeed a moment of staggering achievement and splendour. You can breathe much easier because you are no longer staring at the fear in their eyes. Seeing that fear makes you feel quite a bit shit, which in turn makes them feel shittier, which makes you feel even shittier, and so the cancer circle viciously goes on.

By completing your mission, they feel special AND you feel special.

And you *are*. Special.

You are allowed to feel that way. You are allowed to swagger.

EMBRACE IT

You need to embrace it, remember it and, yes, enjoy it.

Embracing your swagger and being the perfect cancer host can only be positive. Only *you* are in control of how people behave around you and, therefore, only *you* can determine, to some degree, the quality of your social surroundings at this time.

Your best friend's father, a man who used to scare the shit out of you when you were fifteen, might come over to talk to you at a party. You don't look your best. You are puffed up, blotchy and bald. No, you haven't been at the red wine again. You have cancer. He looks slightly terrified at the prospect of having to make conversation and shouts rather manically for his wife to come and rescue him/come and say hello to you. You are in control. You have the status. It was never like this thirteen years ago. He used to bark at you when he was driving you and his children to school. Now, YOU have the status. A few choice words, a softening of the voice, a joke to make them laugh, a couple of self-putdowns and one shared experience recollection later, and they have stopped hyperventilating and walk away feeling good about themselves for having the courage to come and talk to you. You walk away with the knowledge that you used your status for good, not evil.

You don't walk away. You swagger away.

Work that swagger.

This is your moment.

That was my moment.

DERELICTION OF DUTY

It can be confusing having cancer. Really confusing.

It is on your mind all the time.

Of course it is.

Why wouldn't it be?

It would be.

It is.

But it would really help your sanity and your cluster-fuck mind clutter if you could put cancer to the back of your thoughts for just a few moments.

And now and again you can. You do.

Now and again you stop and realise that in those last brief few moments you *have* got on with the task in front of you and forgotten about those little bastards causing havoc inside you.

But therein lies the problem. The longer you forget about it, the harder it is to deal with when you remember it. Not only that, but you feel quite strange about forgetting. Guilty even.

As if you've neglected your best mate in their time of need and crisis. As if you've been a shit friend. You are letting down those people who expect that every waking moment of your life is about '*battling bravely*'. You are letting down those people who believe you should have 100 per cent focus on the job in hand. That job being beating cancer. Any wavering from that is a dereliction of duty. An offence you should be punished for. As if your current punishment isn't enough!

So there you are feeling shit about forgetting that you're feeling shit.

Like I say. It's confusing.

WE ALL NEED AN OJ TRIAL

My attention span isn't what it was. Come to think of it, it never was what it was. Filling time when you are well is one thing. When you have been diagnosed with a life-threatening illness, it's a whole different ball game.

It's an art, in fact.

Having too much time to think is exactly that.

Too much time. To think.

I was lucky when I was ill because I had two things to distract me: the OJ Simpson trial and a gambling addiction.

Annoyingly, because of the time difference between here and the States, prime-time 'OJ live' started pretty much exactly the same time as Napoleons Casino opened. (2 p.m. back then. Now casinos are twenty-four hours.) The casino almost always won. That's how I knew it was an addiction.

The addictive thing about an addiction is that it makes time disappear. It makes twenty-four hours go in a heartbeat. A sweat inducing, adrenaline-filled heartbeat.

Now, I'm not saying that if you get cancer and you don't have an addiction that you are at a disadvantage. And I'm definitely not saying that if you get cancer and you don't have an addiction, get an addiction. I wouldn't dare say that. I would be strung up. By the short and curlies. And seeing as the chemo made every single hair on my body fall out, I didn't have any short and curlies to be strung up by. I do now. You could string me up now. But that's not really the point.

The point is that being immersed in something so deeply – even if it is an addiction – does allow your mind breathing space from the evils of cancer. And that breathing space feels like a positive.

The only problem is that when you are lost in the throes of a gambling addiction, you don't want to breathe. Or have time to breathe, for that matter. And time is money. Time is money won and time is lots of money lost. So the breath from cancer that I so craved was swallowed up by the breathlessness that is gambling. Like I said, it's complex and contradictory.

Contradiction is impossible to avoid. In fact, the very act of writing this book has made me realise how painful and exhausting fighting those contradictions was. And in some ways still is!

The OJ trial was a fantastic distraction. For someone like me who is endlessly fascinated by the vagaries, nuances and, yes, contradictions of human behaviour, watching an obviously guilty man trying to convince the world of his innocence was mesmerising and completely immersive.

And when you have stage 4 sclerosing mediastinal non-Hodgkin's lymphoma, you're not looking for gentle distraction or mild disruption; you're looking for full on diversion immersion.

I do love a mantra. And deep in the heart of cancer and a gambling addiction, a mantra that has nothing to do with either and yet rings around my head so prominently that it forces other thoughts into its recess is a jewel among the shit.

'If the gloves don't fit, you must acquit.'
'If the gloves don't fit, you must acquit.'
'If the gloves don't fit, you must acquit.'

Johnnie Cochrane's trial-winning mantra buried itself in everybody's psyche. Especially mine. And, more especially, the jury's.

Now, I wouldn't go so far as to say I have a mild form of Tourette's. No. But I do sometimes struggle to keep words and phrases in my head. Sometimes they shoot out of my mouth before I even have a chance to suppress them. That's my excuse anyway. Plus, as well as being a mantra lover, I am also a certified flogger of dead horses.

So, here's a bald man with a giant head and a magnificently swollen mouth, walking the streets, chuntering to himself:

'*Gloves don't fit, must acquit.*'

'*Gloves don't fit, must acquit.*'

'*Gloves don't fit, must acquit.*'

I must have scared people shitless. But no matter. It was a magical revitalising medicine all of its own!

The OJ trial was not only an extraordinary piece of theatre, it also became a great excuse to host much needed visitors. I had shunned the idea that I might move back home to my parents' house when I was diagnosed. I knew the only way I could get through this thing was to create a *me* environment. A place I could escape to. A place that would be my own sanctuary of serenity. My futon became my hospital bed, my day unit and my dinner table all rolled into one.

Visiting hours were from 9 a.m. to 9 p.m.

Only visitors bringing satisfactory chocolate-type gifts would be allowed in. M&S microwavable foodstuff would be accepted.

Flowers or anything that needed constant care (apart from me) must be left at the threshold.

And so my visitors *would* appear and they would bring food and chat and watch OJ. It was perfect.

It almost made me forget the cancer and the gambling. Almost.

And almost is joyously better than hardly. These mini miracles were life-saving.

Talking of miracles, on 3 October 1995 the BBC reported the following:

Orenthal James Simpson was found NOT GUILTY of the murders of Nicole Simpson and Ron Goldman... Judge Lance Ito ordered

OJ Simpson to be released 'forthwith' ending 473 days in custody…
Members of the victims' families were distraught: Fred Goldman,
father of Ronald Goldman, said the day of his son's murder was the
worst day of his life, and today was the second.

'I deeply believe that this country lost today. Justice was not served,'
he said.

In a statement, Jason Simpson expressed his father's relief that 'this
part of the incredible nightmare that occurred is over'.

I, on the other hand, had only served half of my cancer sentence.

I was shocked but not surprised by the verdict. I was in mourning for the loss of my OJ trial cancer distraction. I tried to resist the lure of the casino but it had a hold on me stronger than me. It seemed to know that it could comfort me in my OJ trial bereavement. It seemed to instantly latch on to me and recognise my need to fill the OJ void. Gambling smiled at me and beckoned me in, and I was defenceless and unable to resist. I gave in daily to its magnetic charms. I felt weak and fulfilled all at once. Those contradictions robbed me of any strength of will that I may have had left. It felt good. It felt bad.

The forces inside of me were at war. And I was powerless to stop them.

CANCER VERSUS GAMBLING, PART THREE

The fight between cancer and gambling was the heavyweight clash of the titans. I was in the centre of it. It was chain-gang gruelling. They fought for my attention. They demanded that they were the first thing I thought of when I woke up and the last thing I thought of when I fell asleep. They were insanely jealous of my other lover and would constantly raise the bar in order to get more attention. The most painful and confusing thing was that I would constantly use one as respite from the other. They became in turn my best friend and my worst enemy.

There were days when I would arrive in an empty casino at 2 p.m. and it would feel marvellous. Serene, peaceful and calming. It would feel like home. Three hours at a blackjack table would just glide by, and as long as I wasn't winning too much or losing too much it would be the perfect escape. And the croupiers knew me well enough to know that I didn't like to talk. I was just there to play. And it always produced a smile in me when one or two asked what had prompted me to shave all my hair off. This was my thing. My time. Me time. And cancer wasn't allowed in. Casino rules stated: ***Leave your coats and your cancer at the reception desk***. Cancer fucking hated that. Couldn't believe it was being left at the door. For those few hours gambling was stroking me and cuddling me. Gambling was giving cancer the two-fingered salute. And even though it was all wrong, it was all right. I wasn't in my life; I was on some other plane, some other universe. But, of course, the moment you start getting a bit spiritual and hippyish, reality will force your feet back on the ground and slap you hard around the face. Despite being sworn enemies, evil is evil is evil, so if cancer and gambling can collude to make one enormous painful mess then so much the better. And they did. Often.

PRINGLE GUY

I was sitting at the blackjack table in a tunnel of escape and calm when out of the blue someone on my table made a ridiculous call and I lost. And I not only lost that call but I lost my cool and my equilibrium and my karma. And I know now that that person who made the dodgy blackjack move may have looked like just a chain-smoking guy wearing grey slacks and a Pringle sweater, but he was actually sent by the cancer cult to discombobulate me. It's clear that Pringle man was not only working for the cancer cult but for the addiction cult, too. And his ridiculous call led to my veil of rationale being ripped away from me and the red mist instantly descending. In the next five minutes I had zero control over my actions. I loaded each bet with more and more money. And I knew I was going to lose. But I kept loading the bet with more and still more. Self-hatred and self-destruction spewed out of every orifice and I needed to lose. Needed to self-flagellate. Needed to remind myself what a disgusting individual I was. And the addiction cult leader was laughing in my face. And the more he laughed, the more I needed to self-destruct. Until I was empty. Inside and out. And the only thing to do was leave. I picked up my coat and cancer on the way out and made it to fresh air. But the air wasn't fresh and my cancer was ten times heavier than before. Cancer forced itself on me and refused me the big deep breath I craved in that moment. And cancer, too, was laughing in my face. And I was hot and dizzy and nauseous.

Life is shit and I am shit and it doesn't matter which of those will take my life first but please oh please oh please, one of them do it now and do it quick.

Gambling addiction addles your brain. It soaks up everything else until you have pure gambling focus. You get no relief from it. Absolutely none. However, in the battle for total mental preoccupation, gambling has a fierce and all-conquering rival. Cancer. And that's the mind fuck. As an addict, all you're searching for is a single moment of breath. A single moment of thought-free clarity. And that moment almost never comes.

Cancer is ruthless in its pursuit of absolute power. So in the early cancer days, when side effects were minimal, cancer allowed me to storm ahead with the gambling and jog along with the cancer. But jealousy is an ugly old dish best served freezing fucking cold through a giant syringe. And when cancer kicks into action, nothing and nobody can stand in its way. Lying in a hospital bed, unable to speak, feeling like utter shite was weirdly a sort of free-from-gambling breathing space.

And a breath is a breath is a breath. Gambling became a distant memory. For a while. A golden age memory that you yearn for, that makes you feel gooey at the reminiscence but doesn't invade your every pore.

So you see the complexity of the battle.

This wasn't a fleeting skirmish. No. This conflict lasted for pretty much the whole time that I was in cancer mode. And its constancy was totally exhausting.

PESKY-LITTLE-BROTHER-CANCER

There's a whole world out there of people who name their tumours. Like pets. Naming your tumour is all the rage. It's the Steve McQueen of cancer coping. Cool and iconic, I mean. Rather than dead!

Some do it to belittle their tumour and take the edge off its power.

It's an intruder.

It came in without invitation.

If I ignore it, it will make itself at home and decide to stay.

If I name it, I will have control over the bastard.

It is an unwanted guest who needs to be evicted.

It will not control me.

I will name it and then kill it.

From talking to a number of people about this, I learned that naming your tumour is just as tricky as naming your child. Although in this case you don't want it to grow. You want it to shrink. You want your tumour child to shrink.

GERALDINE AND STEVE

While exploring the naming-your-tumour phenomenon, I came across an amazing American called Geraldine who has a brilliant travel blog called The Everywhereist. In one of her blogs she writes about having been diagnosed with a brain tumour (tumor if you happen to be American) and how and why she named it Steve.

The discovery of Geraldine and Steve inspired me to keep

trawling the internet looking for more people who gave their tumour a name. I found hundreds.

These included:

Irving – *shortened to Irv when the tumour shrank*
Abi – *Abi-normal*
Camilla – *It hid like a chameleon*
Bob – *kill Bob and/or Bob was the evil spirit in* Twin Peaks
Itsy and Bitsy – *a multi-tumour name*
The Tumornator – *I'll be back*
Tommy Tumor
Tom – *Tormentor Of Mine*
Rascal
Little Rascal – *it shrank!*
Bugger
Little Bugger – *it shrank!*
PITA – *Pain In The Arse*
OvarianDunWith

These are just the tip of a very large iceberg. It got me wondering how you named a blood cancer rather than a tumour. Was I going to have to spend the rest of my life giving a name to every little evil white cell? Maybe. I spent hours trying to think of witty things to say around this subject. As you might have gathered by now, I often spend hours trying to think of witty things to say. In this instance I drew a blank. But my online search uncovered a man who called his white cell count The Blue Meanies.

According to Wikipedia: 'The Blue Meanies are a fictional army of fierce, if buffoonish, music-hating creatures in the surreal 1968 Beatles film *Yellow Submarine*. They allegorically represent all the bad people in the world.'

Enough said.

In the absence of having a name for my cancer, I would treat it like my annoying little brother. I say brother because I always wanted a younger sister. If I had a younger sister, she would be my best friend, she would not take any of my surly grumpy shit and by now I would have slept with most of her friends.

A younger brother type of cancer is much easier to hate. Much easier to try to ignore. He's the little pest who's growing up far too fast. He has the infuriating habit of wanting to show off when your friends are around. A younger brother type of cancer makes unwanted appearances at inopportune moments. His appearance would manifest itself in a variety of different ways.

On some days I would wake up and feel great. Not just fine. Not just 'feeling OK considering'. But fucking great. It would often be the day *after* chemo. That thrust of oddly coloured liquids pumped into my veins had clearly given me some kind of spurt of adrenaline. Laced with a small shot of euphoria. And it felt surprising. Surprisingly fantastic.

I was a giddy teenager after a first night of passion.

I was Leonardo DiCaprio just before the big boat sank.

I was invincible.

And that's the trap. That's the evil of Pesky-Little-Brother-Cancer.

I would bound out of bed, feeling happy with the world. Feeling happy that I had the ability to bound. When given the opportunity to **bound**, I **bound**. All is good with the world. Today. At this moment.

I would **bound** into the shower. I would **bound** into my ill-fitting clothes.

I'd skip breakfast because breakfast is a bit of a risk. Food tastes shit so I didn't want that reminder to de-**bound** me. I *did* take my six squillion steroids because oddly on good days they didn't symbolise much. Today they were just pills to be consumed. So I scoffed down the pills. I excitedly **bounded** downstairs to get to the outside world.

And the sun's out and it felt good to be out. **Bounding**. And Tufnell Park was the Med that day. No sea or sand to speak of but a great Turkish kebab shop. Which counts. I walked fifty yards to the newsagent. Exchanged pleasantries. I'm always in a better mood on holiday.

I bought a pint of milk, a Diet Coke and the *Guardian*. I returned home, opened the front door and started to ascend the many stairs to my sea-view Tufnell Park Mediterranean penthouse. There were quite a few stairs. Thirty maybe. That's quite a few when you have cancer.

I **bounded** up six of them. Six stairs a-**bounding**. Out of nowhere, my **bounding** was interrupted by a gentle tap on my shoulder. I stopped. Just briefly. Turned. There was nobody there. Weird. I set off on my **bound** again. Once more my **bound** was interrupted by a tap-tap-tap.

This time, it wasn't just a tap on my shoulder, it was in between my eyes, all down my thighs, in the pit of my stomach and deep in my cranium. And I say a tap. It was much more of a punch than a tap.

A long hard, deep full-body punch.

And not just one punch, more of a pummel of punches. A never-ending, stomach-churning, breath-taking pummelling. I slowly turned to face it. Face him. Face it. And this time there WAS someone there.

Staring at me was my bastard Pesky-Little-Brother-Cancer.

He was snarling at me. Bottom lip out. Squealing. He was actually squealing:

I'm still here, you know. You can't ignore me. You're supposed to be looking after me. I'm not looking after you. You're looking after me. I'm your pesky-little-brother-cancer. You can't get rid of me just like that. You can't truly believe that one day you will wake up and I will just be gone.

Just like that. Don't think that if you just ignore me I will disappear. I won't. I will not. If you ignore me, I'll make your life a fucking misery. A misery. I will.

'Don't ignore me. Don't ignore me. Don't ignore me. Don't ignore me. Don't ignore me. Don't ignore me. Don't ignore me. Don't ignore me. Don't ignore me.

'Do Not Ignore Me.

'Do

Not

Ignore

Me.

'Still here. Still here.

Still here.

Still here.

Still here.'

And, despite this terrifying hallway assault, I made it to the top of the stairs. I was just about able to unlock my door. I flopped on my futon/bed/dinner table/self-care unit. I was completely shattered. Physically *and* emotionally. I felt like I had cycled to New York, run the New York marathon and cycled back. In a day.

I peeked out of my top-floor window. The sea and the sand had been replaced by a grey, grim metropolis. My Med penthouse was now a small studio flat above a shop in Tufnell Park. My gaze took me above the shops, beyond the grey and back into my mind again.

Being free of my Pesky-Little-Brother-Cancer seemed like a hazy nostalgic very distant memory. And that's the thing. The whole point.

I *had* successfully managed to ignore him for what seemed like a proper lifetime. A whole hour maybe. A whole fucking hour. Just under. Maybe. Maybe thirty minutes. Maybe less than that. I don't know. But a whole bunch of minutes anyway. And now the miserable, invasive little fucker was back. Big time. And not only would he not go away and not stop reminding me of his presence, but the very fact that I had evaded his grasp for longer than a moment made his reappearance all the more bile-forming and painful. I felt my eyes moisten but I didn't let them cry. Couldn't let them cry. It felt painful now, yes, but at least I was allowed a brief glimpse of the other world. A world of normal that I had struggled to remember. And that brief glimpse was **bound**-making and glorious. And brief.

Too brief. My world had been invaded by cancer. I wanted to be normal. I wanted to be the youngest child again. All I wanted was for my Pesky-Little-Brother-Cancer to fuck off. And die.

But he didn't die. Not for a long while, anyhow. He was right there in the heart of things. Mixing things up. Making those appearances when he was least expected and definitely least wanted. What I'm talking about here is:

Sex. **Sex**. Sex. It's a complex, delicate thing. **Sex**.

At the best of times.

With cancer, it's a whole different ball game. So to speak. As I detailed earlier, the getting to the point where I might partake in sex with another human being didn't seem to be that tricky. The cancer swagger seemed to do all the work for me.

It's one thing to *think* you want sex. It's another to *actually* want it.

I'd find that getting to the point of being just about to have sex was great. Because it's all about the chemistry, the body language, the flirting. And it was familiar territory. It was exhilarating and normalising. I found myself at the point of de-clothing and getting down to the thing. The sex thing. And the adrenaline mixed with the familiarity made me feel wonderfully normal. Wonderfully cancer-free. And the clothes departed and it was skin on skin. That first naked moment with a new partner is an irresistible moment. Thrilling. Deeply sexy. A little bit scary. And sometimes quite magical. Even more stimulating when you have cancer and it's helping you escape. Helping you forget.

But cancer really doesn't like you escaping and forgetting for too long. Hell no. That's not in the fucking rules. What I mean by that is it's not in the goddamn rules. I don't mean it's not in the Rules of Fucking. That's another book entirely! And from nowhere Pesky-Little-Brother-Cancer would rear his poisonous head from under the covers.

'Only me! Don't forget me, you know. You can't forget me, you know. I am going nowhere very fast. Very, very fast. Nowhere fast. Nowhere fast.'

And it's not just a sudden cabin-pressure loss of energy when you least expect it. Though that doesn't help, of course. Having the stamina of a ninety-year-old is not helpful for your sexual prowess, nor is it particularly attractive to your chosen wooing partner. No, Pesky-Little-Brother-Cancer is much cleverer than he looks. He knows that he can get deep inside your mind and haunt your waking being.

'Do you really think you can do the sex thing with me just sitting here in bed with the both of you? Not sure she'll be happy doing it with me watching. With your pesky-little-brother-cancer watching. Not sure it's right. Is it right? Not sure it is really. Have you even told her I exist? Oh yes, that's how you got her into bed in the first place. So you see, without me, you'd be nothing. NOTHING. I can't leave. Won't leave. I am here for the duration. For the ride. If you do want to do it, the sex thing. If you REALLY want to do it, the sex thing, you will have to just pretend I don't exist. Pretend I had never been born. Pretend all is normal. Does she think it's normal? Is she doing it because of the cancer or despite it? Is this normal? Can she see your cancer under your naked skin as she's fucking you? Can she? Can she? Can she? Can she see it? Your cancer. Can she see it and smell it? Your cancer. Me. Your pesky-little-brother-cancer. Me. Is it me she actually wants, not you? Me. Me. Me. Me she wants. Not you. Me. Me. Me.'

Because that's the other thing about Pesky-Little Brother-Cancer. You just can't shut him up. However hard you try. He keeps up a constant stream of consciousness that just bores into your soul.

And Pesky-Little-Brother-Cancer doesn't just bore into your soul. He bores into every particle of your body, soul and mind, too. In fact, Pesky-Little-Brother-Cancer has managed to mess with your mind so chronically that he actually succeeds in planting the thought into your psyche that you could transmit the cancer by doing the sex.

You are there, you are both **almost there**. Almost. Almost there. Just at that moment. Just as you can spot the nirvana of ecstasy and release literally coming around the sexual corner:

'*Only me. Pesky-Little-Brother-Cancer. Just a random thought, nothing to worry about, just a thought to pop into your head at this moment, this moment where you are about to feel a little bit of joy and release for once. Just a thought for you to carry with you on this ride, on this journey. On this doing the sex thing. **What if, what if, what if, what if?***

'*What if this is catching?*

'***What if** just a tiny little orgasm-type moment will infect not just this present partner but the world? The whole world. Your infected seed will escape into the world and a whole new killer epidemic will be released. A "Raz-Cancer-Sperm-release-after-doing-the-sex-thing" epidemic. **What if** you are selfishly sacrificing the whole world for just a tiny bit of happiness? **What if, what if, what if, what if, what if, what if, what if, what if, what if, what if, what if, what if, what if, what if, what if, what if?***'

And then he's gone. And so have you.

And it wasn't just the unexpectedness of his guest appearances that was hard to take, it was the fact that every time I thought I had found some equilibrium, he would turn up to remind me that this wasn't just a moment-to-moment changer, this was a life-changer. Or death-changer.

Pesky-Little-Brother-Cancer didn't just steal the limelight, he did a career-defining, show-stopping nine-month song-and-dance number. And my personality found it hard to keep up. And the 'me me' I was rediscovering began to fade. People stopped seeing me as me. They saw me as Cancer Boy or Alien Boy.

Of course, sometimes he was great to hide behind. It was a relief to have people perceive you in such a defined way. It was curiously uplifting. Having spent twenty-eight years searching, here in one very foul cancer swoop, my Pesky-Little-Brother-Cancer gave me a full, fascinating and detailed personality, with a rich backstory to boot. And it was liberating. And, of course, that's who I was. Most of the time. And most of the time I was indeed happy to banish the elephant and call a cancer spade a cancer spade. On some days Cancer 'me me' was freedom. Real freedom. But some days I longed for people to just see plain old me.

I wanted them to see me.

Not take one look at me and try not to frown.

I wanted them to see me.

Not take one step back before gathering themselves and only then take two steps forward.

I wanted them to see me. Not lower the tone and volume of their voice when they spoke to me.

I wanted them to see me.

Not someone they were impressed by for being so strong and brave.

I wanted them to see me.

Not my Pesky-Little-Brother-Cancer.

Wii CANCER

Hospital can be achingly dull.

To be fair, it's not meant to be a holiday camp. There's a reason why the staff wear white coats more than they do red coats. But even so, being a day patient having chemotherapy or – even worse – being on a ward for days on end can try the patience of a sane person let alone an adrenaline-starved, gambling addicted person. And online gambling wasn't yet a thing back then so I couldn't even distract myself with that. Thankfully.

Nick Hornby was my saviour. Revisiting the brilliant *Fever Pitch* and devouring his new novel, *High Fidelity*, soaked up some of the boredom, but that still left many long hours to be filled. So I resorted to my imagination. I say that slightly disparagingly only because I was often worried that, along with my self-diagnosed academic ineptitude, I didn't quite have the creativity or imagination needed to make it in the arts. It took me a long time to cast aside such insecurities and it was moments such as these – long stretches of hospital nothingness – that helped me reconnect with that side of me.

One of my favourite daydreams was my virtual-reality (I was SO ahead of my time) imaginings of being inside my own computer game and fighting the cancerous aliens inside me. This was 1995. Space Invaders was SO eighties.

THE GAME

- A single-player game.
- Age: 8 to 108.

Object of the game: To terminate your tumour.

How to play:
1. Identify your tumour.
2. Get to know it. Inside and out.
3. Identify its location.
4. Identify its size.
5. Hunt it down.
6. Terminate it.

GAMING ADVICE 1

Always be vigilant. Take nothing for granted:

- The Tumour© has a life of its own.
- The Tumour© may randomly double in size when you least expect it to.
- The Tumour© may lay dormant for any length of time and appear when you least expect it to and in the most unlikely places.

WEAPONS

A) Chemicals
- Identify the right chemicals for the job.
- Track them down.
- Target The Tumour©.

Be aware:
The chemicals also have a life of their own. The chemicals have the capacity to do a 180-degree turn on the spot and attack you as well as your tumour.

B) Radioactivity
- You have access to radioactive zappers that target with pinpoint accuracy the weak spots of The Tumour©.

Be aware:
Radioactive zapping is a long, hard and tedious way of attacking The Tumour©. It requires patience and endurance. It will drastically reduce your energy levels.

HOW TO WIN

This is a game of endurance.

This is a game of perseverance.

This is a game of patience and application.

This is a game of focus and dedication.

- You have nine lives before it's game over.
- Your ability to focus on 'how' to play the game will be continually impeded by your inability to stop yourself wondering 'why' you have to play the game at all and 'if' there will ever be an end to the game.

GAMING ADVICE 2

You are not only fighting The Tumour©, you are also fighting the very weapons you are using to fight The Tumour©!

Be alert at all times.

USER REVIEW

This is a game I didn't want to play but I was forced to. I was given no other choice. I am not a gamer by nature but the object of this game couldn't be simpler. The only drawback is that I have to learn the game at the same time as I am playing the game. There is no trial run.

The game seems to take forever to play. Time passes and I feel calm because I have found some sort of even keel that I didn't think I'd find when I first pressed play. I have no idea whether I am close to winning or not.

As I am solely focused on reducing the size of the evil tumour, I hardly notice how close to the finishing line I am. I keep going. I'm almost there. I reach for the zapper to finish off the little fucker, and out of nowhere and through no fault of my own, The Tumour© turns to face me, does a cartoon skidding halt and mockingly trebles in size. I lose a life and have to start all over again.

There is no worse moment in the playing of this game than this! It feels like I have lost much more than just one life. Everything I'd worked hard for. Gone. All those strategies to move me along in the game were seemingly for nothing. The game makes me feel empty. My insides that were so filled with hope and anticipation and pre-winning euphoria are now just a barren husk. It seems like an almost impossible task to take a deep breath, pick up the game, press go, and start all over again. It would be easier to just give up.

The finishing line is invisible yet it's taunting me. The sound effects on the game seem to have been turned up to eleven and they are whispering:

'You're not going to make it.'

'It's too hard.'

'You're too tired.'

'You will never get to the next level.'

'You're fucked' (it's an adult game).

'Give up.'

The thought of carrying on makes me feel nauseous and exhausted and angry. It would be so much easier just to admit defeat. But the pause button keeps flashing. It's winking at me. And the wink is a glimpse. Or a clue. Or a reminder – that maybe I am not starting from the same point that I did way back whenever. Maybe I learnt more than I think I did when I played the game the last time. And maybe that's the point of this game:

A series of learned responses that will help me get further every time, give me more coping strategies when I have a setback and fill me up with an unexpected amount of confidence and patience that, eventually, may help me make it over the finishing line. And even if I don't quite make it over that line, the very act of playing the game may have afforded me a tiny respite from the insanity of it all.

So all I have to do is press restart and let my instinct and my spirit take over and try to enjoy rather than endure the game. The effort of trying to enjoy it will often feel just that. An effort. But there will be times when I do forget myself and it will feel like I am travelling through the game with ease, maybe even with a certain amount of thrill and pleasure. And that's much more than nothing.

So I press the flashing restart button and begin my next life. That's Wii Cancer. It's just a game.

EMOTIONAL ROULETTE

Cancer does throw up (often literally) a multitude of emotions.

Some obvious. Some completely unexpected. They can appear at any time and are often triggered by the most unlikely of scenarios. You try to fight them but they are bigger than you and often somewhat uncontrollable. Sometimes it is magnificent just to surrender yourself to an emotion and have a spectacularly self-indulgent wallow.

We are allowed to wallow for a small percentage of the twenty-four-hour cycle.

It's in the Cancer Contract.

THE CANCER CONTRACT
You may have an hour of wallowing a day if for the other twenty-three hours you don your Cancer Poncho and square up to the bastard face-to-face.

Too much wallowing leads to guilt. And there's so much guilt flying around already.

- **Guilt** if you're ill:
You think you're a burden. You think that people are putting THEIR lives on hold for you. And you feel guilty about that. But at the same time you have a burning desire to scream out: *'Look after me – take care of me.'*

And sometimes we do ask for help and it feels good, but even when it feels good we feel **guilt** as it seems self-indulgent somehow. So we never scream as loud as we want, and however loud we do scream you know it won't make it better. It just may make us feel a touch better for one brief moment.

And some of your friends are awkward around you and they don't really know how to speak to you and it should be *you* that puts them at their ease but because you feel a bit shit you haven't really got the energy to do so. And you feel terrible guilt about that.

• **Guilt** if it's your loved one who is ill:
You think you are not helpful enough, and anyway why can't it be me that's ill and not them? You'd absolutely swap places if it meant that you didn't have to see them go through this hell.

• **Guilt** for being thankful that it isn't you who is ill:
GUILT GUILT GUILT.
A Jew with cancer! My guilt cup runneth over.

And there is no telling *what* emotions will appear, or *when* they will appear or indeed *why* they will appear.

Random emotional outbursts may occur.

With me, the pressure of being the I at the centre of the emotional hurricane seemed to unlock coping skills I never knew I had. There is an often unspoken expectation from your friends and family that you might be feeling a certain way. They normally expect you to feel worse than you often do, so it's sometimes hard for them to get their head round you being so chirpy. It makes them uncomfortable even.

'*I have steeled myself to be in carer mode. I have practised my bedside manner and my soft, whispery sympathetic voice. I expected you to look like you have cancer. I didn't expect you to be jolly and high-energy and inappropriate. I am not prepared for this! At all!*'

Of course, sometimes we *do* feel shit but we are so adept at hiding it that they are more confused than ever.

My random meltdown moments often happened alone. Sometimes they were not so random. They could easily be explained. It's just that they would appear when I least expected them to.

It was September 1995.

I was replete with mouth ulcers. I couldn't talk, couldn't eat and my white count was lower than the *Titanic*. I wasn't in a good way. Yet my dear friend, the Chairman, was getting wed to the soon to be Mrs Chairman and I really wanted to be there.

September 23rd, the date of the wedding, is etched on my mind. Just four or five days earlier, Oral Armageddon had started. I was being monitored 24/7 and was on intravenous antibiotics that were so strong that the main side effect was a terrifying twenty-four-hour extreme flu symptom cycle.

Freeze, freeze, freeze, boil, boil, boil, extreme boil, extreme freeze, extreme boil, shakes, shakes, shakes, shakes, sweat, sweat, sweat, freeze, freeze, boil, boil, shit, shit, shit.

That was the Thursday. The wedding was on Saturday. It was in Cambridge. I was in London. I wasn't going to make it. Or so everybody thought.

Everybody. Except me.

The doctors were insistent:

'You can't go. You are ill. Very ill. You can't possibly leave hospital, get in a car, travel to a wedding, be at a wedding with a hundred and fifty other people – when your immune system is practically defenceless – journey back to London and return to hospital. You can't do it. Physically you can't do it. You are on an intravenous antibiotic drip twenty-four hours a day. You are seriously ill. Do you hear me? You can't go. You just can't. It's impossible. I'm sorry but you can't go. You can't. You can't.'

Now, forgive my French, but you can't say **can't** to a cunt.

A belligerent, stubborn, truculent, twenty-eight-year-old cancer cunt.

All through my illness people tried. And people failed.

This was one of my closest friends marrying a woman who I adored. I was very ill. I may well have been close to death. Things weren't looking that good. Either as a prognosis or as just my head.

So it was a cancer no-brainer:

If I didn't go and I made a full recovery, I would always regret it. And if I didn't go and ended up dying, well, then, it was clearly pointless not going in the first place.

So **I'm going**.

How I'm going – logistically, physically and emotionally – is a whole other question. But **I am going**. Once the doctors and nurses looked me in the eyes, they knew there was no point trying to stop me.

Because **I'm going**.

I still couldn't really speak because of the ulcers but they understood what I meant:

'Eyer oo ayp meengo oor ayl ichard eysewel.'

Which roughly translated meant:

'Either you help me go or I'll discharge myself.'

My mother wanted to help me. She thought it was crazy that I was intending to go, but she knew me well enough to know she couldn't stop me. She respected me enough not to try. But she wanted to help. Needed to help even. She offered to drive me to Cambridge, wait for me and drive me back. But somehow I persuaded her and myself that I was OK to drive. Myself. To. The. Wedding.

I wasn't OK. But that's OK!

So, armed with a mountain of drugs and with strict instructions to be back at the hospital no later than ten, I set off for Cambridge and the wedding. It was 1995. There was no sat nav. I had a map. I was seriously hoping I didn't get lost as I'm not sure any passer-by could have coped with an alien boy in a suit popping his huge head out of the window and saying:

'*Ud oo ell eee urgh wyee do ner urrch.*'

The last word is church. You can guess the rest.

I arrived at the beautiful little packed village church in surprisingly good time. I really didn't want to attract too much attention. Before I left, in fact, I spent ages wondering about whether wearing a cap would attract or detract attention. I decided on the naked look. Naked head, I mean. Naked naked would probably have attracted some attention.

I tried to sidle in the back somewhere, but incognito is a bit of a no-no when you've got lots of friends in the church and most of them haven't seen you since you were diagnosed. When they did see me, and saw me looking this bad, however hard they tried to hide it they couldn't conceal the sadness in their eyes. Some of them were lost for words. I tried to overcompensate by doing all the talking but my talking wasn't talking. It was gargle-mumbling. If I wanted to be understood, I had to articulate and the act of articulation made me wince because it involved my tongue having to work too hard and, by doing so, knock against the remaining ulcers. So the words that I spoke were followed by an involuntary wincing, which only served to make the people that I was trying to make feel *less* uncomfortable, feel *more* uncomfortable. So much for incognito! Sitting down and shutting up was now the best bet. Before I properly upstaged this wedding. I found a nice spot next to my welcoming friend Caroline and I just nodded at people with my incognito shiny '**I'VE GOT CANCER. I'VE GOT CANCER**' bald head.

And it was a beautiful wedding. And I do have an annoying tendency to choke up at tick-box weddings. And I guess this wedding ticked more boxes than most. And, true to form, my emotions didn't take long to rise to the surface. The Chairman taking his vows and his voice cracking slightly was all it took to make my stomach churn, my mouth ulcers throb and my tears flow. And I wasn't crying out of self-pity, or anything like that. It was tears of pure unadulterated happiness for them and tears of relief that I was belligerent enough to force myself off my hospital bed, into a car and make it here to see this.

But those aren't the tears I am here to talk about. Those were good tears. Those were '*wash away the pain of now and the pain of mouth ulcer*' tears. The tears that I am talking about come at the end of this overwritten true story.

The wedding was perfect. Nobody expected me to stay for long beyond the ceremony. Least of all me. Maybe just the drinks bit rather than the sit down and eat bit as well. The attention I got at the reception was lovely. It was just what I needed at this pretty horrific stage in the journey. A reminder that all was normal beyond the Marsden walls and the world hadn't run away from me. Life really does go on and, more than that, I don't have to sprint to catch up, I just have to be present. If I am present in whatever form, even in my alien boy/elephant man form, I can click my heels and be back in the game.

So I made it to the drinks and decided I would stay for some of dinner. My hospital curfew was ten. They were absolutely adamant that it could be no later than ten. Later than ten and it was a danger to me. I had to be dripped with antibiotics, monitored and steroided (I made up a word!). The whole nine chemo yards. So no later than ten then. It was roughly 7.30 p.m. when we sat down to eat. There was a woman sitting to my left. I hoped she was nice. She needed to be nice. I wasn't at my small-talk best.

Her opening line was a good one: '*Hi, have you got cancer?*'
'*Uhu.*'
'*I am just recovering from a nervous breakdown.*'
'*Uhu.*'
Holy shit.
She quickly realised that my ability to speak was hindered

by my physical inability to open my mouth without wincing audibly. Plus, if I tried to talk too much, there was dribbling. So my nervous breakdown friend to the left talked to me while I mumbled and nodded and dribbled wittily.

WHAM RAP

It was 9.46 p.m. I was supposed to be back at the Marsden by 10 p.m. I was in Cambridge. The Marsden is in south-west London. I had fourteen minutes to make a journey that would take seventy-five minutes in a Ferrari. I didn't have a Ferrari. I had a Honda Civic. I'd better go. At the very moment that I was mumbling and spitting a goodbye to breakdown woman, I heard a strange calling from the direction of the DJ. It took me a while to work out what it was. It was camp. It was high camp and high tempo. Just up my street! It was Wham! Tune! It was one of my 'stay-alive' songs. It was a sign. Before I leave, I must dance.

Cancer boy busting out his moves. Woo hoo!

'Take me to the edge of heaven, tell me that my soul's forgiven.'

And there I was twirling with the world. For one brief moment I had got my mojo back. My me back. The newly crowned Mrs Chairman got a twirl, the Chairman's mum got a twirl, the Chairman's granny got a twirl, the formerly unhinged woman next to me got a twirl, even the Chairman got a twirl. Talk about stealing the limelight for a moment. And it felt fucking good. More than that it felt releasing and liberating. It felt like freedom (pardon the Wham! pun). If I was going to go, this was how I wanted to go. And I don't mean go in terms of leaving the wedding!

Having said that, it was now about 11.30. I was awash with adrenaline as well as the vast amount of pills (prescription) I had been taking and I really did have to leave. I didn't want to. I could have stayed all night. Could have danced all night! And still have begged for more! But I had to go.

A lot of people were really surprised that I had made it down to Cambridge on my own, let alone was going to drive back up late at night as well. Especially after all that Whamtastic dancing and very little food! To me that seemed fine. I was in my car. I was in control. I was fine. I was maybe a bit sweaty and breathless but I had taken all my pills and I was good to go. There was much consternation and offers of lifts and all sorts but I needed to do it alone. For me. For my soul. For my independent spirit. So I mumbled my goodbyes and left.

HONDA CIVIC MAGIC CARPET

The two-hour car journey back to my new temporary abode was a glorious ride on a rickety old Honda Civic magic carpet. I was floating my way to The Marsden Hotel having sipped from the euphoric glass of **normality**. I had sipped it. I had bathed in it. I had danced with it. I had realised for the first time in almost three months that it wasn't out of my grasp. Just the opposite in fact. And for one brief moment, I had crystal clarity. I had an epiphany. Not a big one or a religious one. A little one. A mini epiphany.

MY MINI EPIPHANY

Floating along the M11, I realised that the wedding was made even more special for me by the condition I was in. My senses and feelings had been opened and heightened by dealing with cancer on a day-to-day basis. Oddly but rather wonderfully, my situation was allowing me to make discoveries about myself and the world that I could never have made without this illness. Wending my way to hospital at God knows how early in the morning, that felt like an extraordinary and perversely magical contradiction. It felt like an epiphany.

If my journey through this thing was as much about trying to discover what's different and special and unique about life as it was about actually getting well, then the one would probably take care of the other. And that seemed like my most positive thought ever! It also meant that I could get lost in the discoveries rather than always having to think about the illness.

And it's not such a radical new thought, but it did feel like an epiphany because it appeared to me with such overwhelming clarity. And that clarity felt truly invigorating amidst the absurdity of the chemo mayhem. That mini epiphany also allowed me to breathe a little easier. Maybe the next chapter wasn't going to be as difficult as the last? Maybe I was close to overcoming one of the many giant hurdles? Only about eighty-four mouth ulcers left to kill.

And in the claustrophobic bubble of my silver Honda Civic at 1.30 in the morning, tears started streaming down my face for the second time that day. These were gentle tears. Almost imperceptible tears. Warm tears. Cynicism-free tears. Comfortable '*I can breathe a bit easier*' tears. These were important tears, but even these are not the tears I am here to tell you about. These were journey tears. Tears along the way tears.

HOME IS WHERE THE HOSPITAL IS

I arrived back at the hospital at 2.45 a.m. Almost five hours late. In disgrace. Well, I say 'disgrace'. The transgressor in me wanted to be shamed and shunned by the whole of the Marsden community. I wanted so badly to hear the words:

'*What time do you call this, young man? You're grounded till further notice.*'

I sauntered into the ward. I had the look of a surly eight-year-old schoolboy. I looked the nurses straight in the eye. My head was cocked provocatively to one side and my eyebrows were raised as if to say:

'Yeah, go on then, punish me, do it, see if I care.'

Instead all I got was a cheeky *'tutt, tutt, tutt'* from the duty nurse. I think he was from New Zealand. He was the most composed, most patient and kindest man you can ever imagine. Looking after me, he needed to be. I can't remember his name. I want to call him Simon. He seemed like a Simon. He's a Simon.

Simon (feels right) had my mountain of medication armed and ready to go. To this day, I remember how calm and sweet and gentle he was. Calm, sweet, gentle Simon. The drugs took about fifteen minutes to administer and then he gently but firmly (that's a good combo!) demanded that I go to sleep. And I did. I went straight to sleep. Fast, sound, cancer-free sleep.

And the next morning instead of a continuation of last night's euphoria, I awoke to find something strange alongside me. I was lying next to an ice cold body with a lifeless heart.

I didn't recognise it at first but slowly it dawned on me.

It was me.

Was it? Am I here? Or did I die? That's it, I must have died. That's it, I had died and yesterday was but a mere last-breath dream. Or even worse, I was still alive. I was still a patient. And I was still ill. Very ill. Nothing had changed. Nothing at all. Nothing was special. Nothing was unique. Just the opposite in fact. The magic carpet had dumped me back here and pushed my face firmly back into the grim dirt of reality. This hellish hospitalised reality. Despite the positivity of yesterday, despite the hope of yesterday, despite the epiphany of yesterday, today I was back in hell. Or worse, living purgatory.

I flat-lined the morning, desperately trying to fuel myself on yesterday's memory. That almost worked. Almost. But not quite. Gradually the early morning darkness gave way to a numbing void. I was staring into space feeling frozen and empty. And just as I was contemplating the longest Sunday in the universe, the most beauteous thing happened. The ward door was flung open and eight of my closest friends arrived. Almost literally straight from the wedding.

Surprise!

A post-wedding Sunday afternoon party!

I'M NORMAL

My gnarly little heart exploded. The darkness vanished. The seven-year-old me demanded all the sweets in the store. All at the same time.

I ate my friends up with the voracity of a fucking raptor. The 'afternoon after the night before' went by in a flash. The wedding had shed all the awkwardness some of my friends had had about confronting my condition.

Today, I was normal. For a couple of hours at least, I was more normal than something really, really normal.

And we chatted around my bed, wandered around the hospital, visited the café – which was '*rather OK for a hospital café*' – returned to the ward, laughed, chatted, reminisced, chatted, laughed. Did I mention we laughed? And because they were my friends (my friends who'd witnessed me dancing like a crazed fucker the night before), who got it, and got me, I didn't need to do too much of the talking. Thank fuck. As it was pretty painful. Talking, that is. They were happy to just chat and chat and chat. However, the longer the afternoon went on, the chattier I became. The pain had all but disappeared. For that one afternoon only, I was ulcer-free. And pain-free. And chemo-free. And cancer-free. I was invincible.

I am immune to reality. My bubble can't be burst. I am floating on a sea of calm and chat and joy and laughter and hysteria. Calm AND hysteria. That's got to be a cocktail everybody needs to try. It is my drug of choice. I immerse myself in it to the utter max. This euphoria of normality MUST NEVER end. It will not end. It doesn't get better than this, right? It can't.

And just as I was surfing a wave higher than I ever imagined possible, the words that I knew were coming, came. I thought that if I talked forever without a breath that somehow, somehow those words wouldn't ever appear.

Those words, man. Those words. Those fucking words.

'Look, Raz, I think we need to take off in a few minutes.'

'Yes, us too, sadly.'

'Shit, is that the time? Where did it go? Us too, I'm afraid.'

Ignore it, Raz. Ignore it. Ignore it. Ignore it. Keep on floating. Embrace your ecstasy. You are pain-free. You are cancer-free. Be entertaining. Be funny. Be inappropriate. Be entertaining, funny and inappropriate and they may stay. Continue being 'fuck-you, cancer' and they may not leave. They may cancel all their arrangements forever and this moment will linger and linger and linger forever. It will not fade into the nothingness of just a memory. Be all those things and more and they will stay and this euphoria will stay and today will stay and tomorrow will never ever come.

But they didn't stay. They began to gather up their coats and bags and stuff. Their slow procession to the exit had begun. And even that was part of the exquisiteness of this moment because they were all genuinely pleased they'd come (I don't think it was necessarily their number-one choice of venue for a hungover Sunday afternoon) as they could see how much it meant to me.

They would walk away from the hospital with a vicarious swagger.

STAY BRAVE

And my face stayed brave during the goodbyes as I knew it was really important to show them how genuinely grateful I was that they had come and how much it meant to me. I am not good at doing any of that stuff, even now, so when I do remember to do it, I do it hard! And I didn't want anything to sour their memory of this moment. I wanted it to be as special for them as it was for me. So I knew it was my job to enable them to leave on a bit of a floating vibe, too. And any chink in my exhilaration would put a chink in theirs and I wouldn't let that happen. So I did my job and sparkled till the last.

And then they were gone. They were gone and the silence was thunderous.

But the post-show glow still remained.

I sat on my bed in peaceful silence with the rest of the ward a blur and reflected on the beauty of the last thirty-six hours. I had defied my own odds, defeated the mighty force of the oncologists, broken a few rules, made it to the wedding, made it out of the wedding, been simultaneously told off and looked after by Nurse Simon (still feels right) and hosted my own wedding comedown party. Not bad for ailing alien cancer boy.

SQUEEZE

And as I was patting myself on the back reflecting on the wonderful oddness of life, I felt a hand begin to slide gently through the pit of my stomach. It crept slowly through my torso, twisting as it went. I knew exactly what was going on but I was powerless to stop it. The hand slithered further and further up my body until it calmly but firmly took hold of my throat and began to squeeze. I couldn't even begin to fight it. It was too forceful. Too intent. Too direct. I had lost any strength I thought I had. It began to squeeze harder and harder until I almost couldn't breathe. I could breathe enough to stay alive but not enough to not want to die. And as I sat on my bed, the hospital ward exploded. A gallery of grotesques sat staring at me and laughing at me and ridiculing me. This seemed to go on for more than ever. I slowly realised I had become the one thing I never wanted to be. A cliché. The hand had me in the uncontrollable grip of loneliness. I was alone. And only clichés were there to keep me company. I alone was fighting this illness and, despite everyone around me wanting to try and be there and be helpful, they couldn't help me in moments like this. It was just me and my clichés. This was a prison with an indefinite sentence. This man was an island. I was back on a lonely road to oblivion. My friends were out in the world now, choosing to do whatever they were choosing to do. And I was here, in the midst of this lunacy. In a world of pain. Alone. And riddled with cancer and clichés.

REFUSE THE TEARS

And it was late Sunday afternoon. And late Sunday afternoons always feel a bit shit. And this aloneness that was gripping my throat gradually extended to every fibre of me. And it was choking me. It's the oddest kind of loneliness. Like you're crawling through the Sahara on your hands and knees with no water and nobody around for miles and miles except a tiny screen in the corner of the sky that is showing you how beautiful and cool and charmed everybody else's life appears to be.

And for the first time since I was diagnosed, I just wanted it all to end. It wasn't special. *I* wasn't special. At all. I didn't want to cope. The pain was irresistible and all-consuming. Tears didn't seem enough for this moment. I refused the tears. Which made the pain even more concentrated. The pain swirled around inside me, prodding and pushing my skin till I felt like an inflated space hopper.

At any moment I will burst and little bits of me will be scattered around the Marsden ward and it will be all over and that can only be a good thing because this pain is too much, and however tough

I thought I was and however much I preach the word of enjoying cancer, this pain disproves all of that and shows me to be the cancer fraud I never thought I was.

And then the tears came.

I had ordered them to stay away but they came anyway. Of their own accord. And they weren't tears, they were oceans and they thrashed against my aching bones and started to drown me. And I didn't fight it. I knew I didn't have the strength. And anyway drowning would end the pain and that can only be a good thing. But they wouldn't stop. The tears wouldn't stop. And the pain wouldn't stop. And the choking wouldn't stop. I managed to pull myself together enough to phone Paul – him from the Paris shower shampoo story. Paul had just been here this afternoon and, quite frankly, he is one of the greatest. And he listened to the wailing and the grief and the self-pity and the clichés, and he said all the right things and just let me verbally vomit it all out. The wrenching vomit seemed to release the grip. Not totally. But enough to allow me to take back a modicum of control.

When I put down the phone, I could at least breathe a bit. Just a bit. The pain was still enveloping but it had left just a tiny bit of room. A tiny bit of room for me to try to get me back. And I took to my bed and the calm gently began to resurface. And the calm very slowly led to a renewed feeling that can only be described as joy. Joy that an addict feels when they admit to themselves that they have hit rock bottom and the only way forward now is forward.

I could breathe and I was certain that I would never feel pain as bad as that again. I was certain that I had dealt with the worst and beaten it down. I had no idea what was to come but I did know that, whatever it was, after this moment I probably had the strength and the insight and the breath to deal with it.

And some sort of serenity after the epic, emotionally charged storm began to emerge. And what does a person most need at such a time?

Golf.

That's right, I said golf.

Ryder Cup golf to be precise.

The Ryder Cup at Oak Hill, Rochester, NY, to be totally exact.

I loved the golf. Still do. Funny but true. Especially the Ryder Cup. It entrances me. The Ryder Cup is escape in its purest and most brilliant form. And it's 1995 and Europe have started to be really good. And it's a team of champions. The beautiful Seve, the not so beautiful but ever heroic Monty, the cunty but brilliant Nick Faldo, and that cheeky old dog from Largs, Sam Torrance.

For those of you who haven't a clue what I am talking about right now, shame on you.

And that was the other worst thing about being in hospital over this weekend. I was going to miss the Ryder Cup. And at this precise moment it wasn't just about the golf itself, it was about a need for a distraction of distinction on the scale of gambling or the OJ trial. My genius mum had a plan. She went out and bought me a little mini earphone AM radio thingy. Now, these days there are so many devices and apps I could find to listen to it with, but twenty-odd years ago there wasn't much choice, and a little mini earphone AM radio thingy was as good as anything.

And so I took to my bed.

Just as that calm was resurfacing, a new pain was rising. The pain of Ryder Cup anxiety. I lay there and magically got lost in the golfing ebb and flow. And I was transported once again. It was going to go right down to the wire. Seve lost his match, but Ryder Cup King Monty, cunty Nick and big Sam all won. There was just enough time for one final cliché on this momentous day. It was time for an unsung hero to bring the cup home.

When Jay Haas missed his putt on the 18th, Philip Walton *was* that hero and in Rochester, NY, the European Ryder Cup team exploded with elation and relief.

Three thousand four hundred and sixty miles away at 1 a.m., in his bed at the Royal Marsden Hospital in South Kensington in London, a young alien cancer boy released his final outburst of emotion for the weekend. An outburst so loud and impulsive that it not only woke up half the fellow patients on his ward but induced more than one nurse to come running to his bedside to see what was wrong. Nothing was wrong. The European Ryder Cup team had defied the odds and won.

And after the tumultuous cliché-packed weekend cancer boy had had, he felt ready, willing and much more able to do the same.

RATION THE RELATIVES

Having my amazing friends come and see me after the wedding and my unexpectedly emotional response to their leaving made me realise something fundamental. If I don't want to see a particular person when I'm fit and healthy, do I want to see that particular person when I am in a hospital bed with a life-threatening illness? No. Thank. You.

Listen up!

If you are thinking of going to visit someone in hospital, think long, think hard:

1. Are you close? By that I mean, are you actually close? **Think long and think hard**. Is **Ill Person** someone you hang out with on a regular basis? By that I mean, is **Ill Person** someone you **actually** do hang out with on a regular basis?

2. If **Ill Person** is a relative, is he/she someone you look forward to seeing on family get-togethers, or is he/she someone you dread being left alone in the same room with? **Think long and think hard**.

3. What does **Ill Person** *really* think about you? This is the moment to have a real proper look at yourself. **Look long and look hard**. Are you looking? Imagine what **Ill Person** might actually think if they knew you were coming to visit. Go on, really think about it. Be honest now. Will they dread it? Will they? Is the answer a big fat yes and you just can't admit it?

4.   Every family has a nightmare relative. Are you the nightmare relative? **Think long and think hard**. Is it you? It IS you, isn't it! Face it! If you want to show compassion, if you want to show **Ill Person** that you are thinking of them, DON'T VISIT. That's a ton of compassion right there.

If you answer the wrong way to most of the above questions, tell **Ill Person** that you are thinking of them. Tell them you were thinking of visiting them but you thought better of it. You thought **Ill Person** would appreciate some peace and quiet. Then you're quids in. You have outed yourself as a nightmare but in the same breath shown you are blessed with self-awareness. You, the nightmare, have made yourself feel good and you have made **Ill Person** feel good too. By not coming. Good job!

Even if you're not the nightmare, your prime reason for visiting **Ill Person** should be for *them*, not for you. That's a really complex consideration and not easily defined. It's like giving someone a present. We give someone a present because we want to make someone happy. The happier we make them, the better we feel about ourselves so inevitably we get quite a bit of reflected glory from it. If we give that person a present and they love it but they don't say so and don't say thank you, does it take the shine off it somewhat? I think it does. It probably shouldn't, but it does. Because we are not given the gift of gratitude and we haven't been granted the opportunity to be puffed up by the knowledge that we have been generous and made someone else happy.

So when you are thinking of visiting – more to the point, when **you** think **you** want to visit – just stop for a moment and consider if your visit will make **Ill Person**'s day better. If you truly think the answer to that question is yes, then do it. Make that visit.

Of course, you might be delusional. A lot of us are. You

might believe that you don't *need* to think about whether you would make **Ill Person** feel better by visiting them because you *know* that you will. When the truth is **you won't**.

And of course delusional people don't know they're delusional, otherwise they wouldn't be delusional.

So if you're reading this and you have thought about it and think: '*Yes, my visit will make* **Ill Person** *feel better,* **definitely**,' you may be delusional or have delusional tendencies, so think again. And again. If the answer's still yes, then you are either blessed with self-awareness or you aren't. I can't be sure. Nor can you. But **Ill Person** knows. Oh yes. **Ill Person**'s heart either sinks or soars when you walk up to their hospital bed.

Look hard at **Ill Person**'s smile. Is it fake? Is it forced? If you think it is, don't stay for long. That's all I'm saying. I wouldn't dream of accusing you of being delusional. Just don't stay for longer than a minute.

If you walk up to **Ill Person**'s bed and they don't even crack a slight smile, it is a good sign. It often means that **Ill Person** is indeed really happy to see you. You are someone they feel comfortable with. Someone they don't feel they have to fake a smile for.

Of course, sometimes a frown means a frown. Sometimes a frown means '*NO, NO, I can't believe you have visited me and I sure am not going to make any effort to hide my disdain*.'

It's a complex thing. Visiting etiquette.

When I was playing the part of the **Ill Person,** my rule was always that I didn't want anyone visiting me who I felt I had to make any kind of effort with. Doing cancer takes enough effort as it is; I didn't need to be forced to make more effort than I had to.

Sometimes, however, in the role of **Ill Person**, it makes *you* feel good if you make the person visiting you feel good. The knowledge that that particular visitor had to force every fibre of their being to face up to this cancer thing that you have in order to come and visit you is often humbling. They were backer-offers who fought themselves and didn't, in the end, back off. You might not be certain that that's the case but you can detect it and, when you do, it feels good. Of course, that soon wears off if that visitor is an absolute fucking bore.

And as the **Ill Person**, there's one skill you need to really perfect: how to make your visitor leave without making them feel too shit.

HOW TO MAKE YOUR VISITOR LEAVE WITHOUT MAKING THEM FEEL TOO SHIT

It's only natural that a visitor brimming with delusion will force you to come up with a cunning exit plan for them. A wanted visitor either knows the right to time to say adios or is quite happy for you to tell them directly. And that's the point. It's just easy. And that's all **Ill Person** wants. Ease.

Sleep is a fine 'please leave' tactic that has been applied successfully for hundreds of years. It works like this:

The unwanted visitors arrive. (**Delusionals** don't hunt alone. They need a companion to egg them on and confirm their delusion to.)

Ill Person is lying on the bed.

The **Delusionals** sit too close to the bed and are drivelling on about some inane nonsense or other.

Ill Person is fake smiling but has zoned out years ago.

Ill Person closes their eyes.

Ill Person mumbles in an incoherent and ill way.

Ill Person tosses a bit. **Ill Person** turns a bit.

Ill Person allows the mumbling to gradually disappear.

Ill Person starts to heavy breathe a bit.

The **Delusionals** are still droning on.

The **Delusionals** stop droning on. Eventually.

Ill Person can feel the **Delusionals'** stale breath far
too close.

The **Delusionals** are still invading **Ill Person**'s ill space.

*'He can't keep his eyes open, poor thing, shall we go? We should
go. Um... ER... ill person, ill person, we are going now, we're
gonna go. So... Hope you feel better... erm, enjoy the grapes and
the word puzzle book thing... erm... bye, ill person... we're off...
bye, ill person. Bye.'*

Ill Person times it perfectly. Just as the **Delusionals** have
turned for the door, **Ill Person** mumbles in a semi-sleep voice:
'Bye... thanks for the grapes and the word puzzle book thing.'

⇓

THE **DELUSIONALS** EXIT HOSPITAL LEFT

And they've gone and you managed to exit them without making
them feel too bad. What am I saying? They're delusional, they
don't feel bad at all. They feel great.

The irony is that when you have 'wanted' people to visit,

you can genuinely fall asleep and it isn't awkward at all. In fact, ironically, what you want is to be able to fall asleep for as long as you need to and your visitor still to be there when you wake up. And you not to feel guilty that you have fallen asleep on your visitor. While you're asleep, your wanted visitor will happily read a magazine, go out and make a phone call, have a cigarette, have a coffee, have a wank, even pop out for a walk and come back. And wait till you wake up. Your wanted visitor knows that you want him/her there when you wake up. **Delusionals** take sleep as an affront. It's a sign that they should leave. So they sort of do know that they're not wanted. They are **Delusionals** in denial!

BACKER-OFFERS

Conversely, there are friends who you want to be close to you at this time but who for whatever reason can't deal with it and just back off. I had a close friend at the time who was one of the first people I told about my diagnosis. I phoned her on her mobile. She was driving. I said she should pull over as I wanted to tell her something and I didn't want her to be driving when I told her. She pulled over. And I told her. Unusually for me, I was fairly joke-free about it.

I told her I had cancer. A thing called non-Hodgkin's lymphoma. A cancer of the lymph glands.

I told her that the doctor had said that if you were going to get cancer, this was a good one to get.

I told her that the survival rates are good. Seventy to 80 per cent.

I told her not to worry.

There was a long silence on the end of the phone.

Followed by audible sobs.

She told me that she didn't know what to say.

She told me that if I needed anything, she was here for me.

She told me that if anybody was made to beat this thing, it was me.

There were more sobs.

She told me to take care. She told me she loved me. She hung up.

I didn't hear from her again for over two years.

I make no judgement. I understand. I really do. People back off. They do. It can be somewhat disappointing. And sad. But that *is* life.

Even my mother had one or two of her friends who didn't quite know how to deal with me being ill or how to talk to her about it. They went silent. Rather than have to confront their own discomfort. She found that odd. She also found it a bit sad. And it *is* a bit sad. But it's also very human. It is too much for some people. They feel so out of their depth that to retreat is the only option. I honestly don't think they know they are doing it.

When someone that we love spending time with – and we feel would be a tonic at a time like this – retreats rather than comes forward, we can't help but feel confused, frustrated and a little bit betrayed. We can't. But we also mustn't let it fester. We have to remind ourselves that some of those people have probably been sitting at home agonising about how best to get in contact. And it's paralysing them. To such a degree that they end up doing nothing. The nothing they are doing is eating them up with guilt.

I heard about numerous people who wanted to send a card to me but didn't because they had wrestled for ages to find the right thing to say. And couldn't. So they eventually gave up. Which is understandable.

It is easy to think that in these circumstances there are right words and wrong words. There aren't. Any words will normally do. Just the knowledge that you have glanced a thought my way is enough. So the '*I don't know what to say*' notes and the

'*I have no words*' notes are just as comforting as something more eloquent.

Of the cards I did get, I particularly liked those which used some kind of gambling metaphor.

'My money's on you.'

'You're a sure bet for recovery.'

They took my addiction and threw it right back in my cancer face. Now *those* are my kind of people!

Dealing with other people and visitors when you're ill is indeed a complex and often challenging thing. You do have to take care of the carers sometimes. It's part of your job. And it *is* complex.

For instance, no matter how open you try to be or want to be when you are ill, no matter how inclusive you are, it seems really wrong and selfish sometimes to tell people of the loneliness that is eating away at you. I don't exactly know why. Someone has put themselves out physically and emotionally to come and see you while you are sick. This might be one of the hardest things they have done in a long time. Every fibre of their being was telling them that they couldn't face it. It was too hard. They longed to back off. But, they fought that particular battle with themselves and won. They made it here. By your cancer bedside. They feel good about themselves for doing so. For wrestling with their own taboos. And facing up to them. To you. When they make it to your bedside, **you** tell them that you feel singular and alone. Well, thanks for that. They love to hear that their visit hasn't helped you one jot. Great. Fucking great. They leave feeling really shit about themselves for being unable to make you feel even a tiny bit better. Brilliant!

And so you spend a lot of energy creating an environment in which the people you want visiting you feel comfortable enough to actually visit. And sometimes the act of a person pushing past their desire to back off and uncomfortably finding themselves by your bedside not quite knowing what to say is not annoying at all but actually beautiful and replenishing.

Two such people were Carla and Katie.

Carla I knew better because we'd had a brief work fling about a year before all this cancer stuff happened. Katie was also someone I worked with. Katie was strange. I quite liked strange. Katie and Carla were friends.

The first time I had been admitted to hospital was a dark time. Confusing. I didn't want to be there. Everything about it was bizarre and uncomfortable. I was in a ward. I was surrounded by ill people. The place stank of illness. I didn't want to be there. Did I say that already? I hadn't quite yet figured out how to be in that kind of environment.

I shall grimace, I shall cry. I shall sulk. That is how I shall be.

It was 3 p.m. I was dozing on my bed. I grimaced as I dozed. I had my clothes on. I wasn't going to wear pyjamas. It was daytime, for fuck's sake. I was dozing and sulking. I opened my eyes. There were two figures at the end of the bed. There was some kind of gel over my POV movie lens. I was in a doze and now I am in a haze. It was a classic post-doze-haze! It took quite a while for the haze to dissolve.

The two figures at the end of my bed were standing side by side, very close together. Facing me. They were smiling nervously. They were holding stuff. I didn't focus on them as I was distracted by the stuff they were holding. The stuff seemed to be a pineapple, a box of Terry's All Gold and a small rather scabby potted plant.

They were smiling even harder now. And then it clicked. **Carla and Katie.**

They both sort of started to talk at once. Sort of repeating each other. They were looking more at each other than they were looking at me.

They said they didn't know whether to come or not. **Didn't**

know. They said they didn't know what the right thing to do would be. **Right thing.** To. Do. **Would be.** They said they were worried about me being notoriously grumpy. **Grumpy.** I wouldn't want to see them. **Wouldn't want to see us.** They said they didn't know. Didn't know. **If.** They would. They. **Know the right thing to say.** Say. So just in case. Case. They brought. A pineapple. **Pineapple.** A pot plant. **Plant.** From Katie's squat. **Squat.** And an unopened. **Unopened.** Box of Terry's All Gold. **Gold.**

They smiled. They laughed. I laughed. It was brilliant. It was perfect. It made me cry. In a good way. Relief for people who got it. Who got me.

And, thankfully, there were more of these great visitor experiences than there were delusional visitors.

In the summer of 1995, I had a '**Champagne and Strawberries Wimbledon Finals Party**'. It was unlike any other. I'm sure of it. This may have been the only '**Champagne and Strawberries Wimbledon Finals Party**' that year to take place in a side room of a cancer ward in a cancer hospital in south-west London. I like to think so anyway. I am not one for parties but this one was impromptu, joyful and unique. People arrived. They brought a Fortnum's hamper with real food that I could almost taste. A picnic was had on my hospital lawn, aka my bed. Tennis was watched, strawberries were eaten, champagne was quaffed (by visitors and a few nurses!) and life seemed surreally beautiful. My non-delusional visitors made it so. A Wimbledon Finals Cancer party. Perfection. Apart from Boris losing, of course.

Same time next year? I hope not.

FUCK GRAPES, GIVE ME TASTE

By the way, where does this idea come from that the thing that will perk us up when we are feeling like shit, looking like shit and have a mouth tasting like metallic shit is grapes? Or any other bland tasteless fruit-type thing that will sit next to our bed, cluttering up our bedside table until they discolour and then rot.

Symbolic, eh! I think that's why people are scared to throw them away. They don't want the death and burial of the said fruit to be misconstrued as a sign of our impending doom!

No!

What we want is food to glory in, food that transports us, food that is so rich and deep in flavour that it wins the fight against metallic-mouth-mania and allows us to forget for a brief moment the constant giddy nausea that we have had to learn to live with for so long.

MORE FLAVOUR. NOT LESS.

That's the only possible chance we have of not being reminded every time we take a mouthful of anything, that the thick killer chemicals that are being pumped into us on a weekly basis have gloried in systematically trying to destroy our taste buds.

Oranges are not the only fruits.

No.

Grilled pesto chicken sandwich with caramelised onions on a toasted ciabatta with triple-cooked chips on the side are the only fruits.

Fuck yeh!

BRAVERY IS

'Battling cancer bravely' is an oft-used phrase.

When I was going through it, I neither thought I was brave nor did I feel as if I was in a battle. But that's not to say I wasn't. It's just not what it feels like to be amidst it. In some ways it feels the opposite of those things. You have no choice.

If I put you on a raft in the middle of the Atlantic with a paddle in your hand and the tiniest glimpse of land in the distance, you could choose to do nothing and drift till the elements took you to oblivion or you could choose to paddle. Bit by bit. You don't know whether you'll make it but you know that you have to try. And you know that if you are moving closer to your destination, then, despite your ever-increasing exhaustion, you have a good chance of actually reaching terra firma. And that possibility means that you unthinkingly keep going. Sometimes you might even go backwards a bit. Those are the moments where you almost literally sink or swim. But, again, the steel in you rises, unwittingly sometimes, and you continue on.

And you don't always make it. Not everyone does, sadly. But you find life and experience and soul in the very act of doing it. And that is 'battling' and that is 'bravery'; it's just normally not conscious and normally not a choice. And over the years since my illness I have seen it time and time again from afar and with people I am close to. And not just with cancer but with all sorts of illnesses and sometimes tragic situations. And my admiration for those people knows no limits.

And so if I were pushed for a definition it would be this:

Bravery is embracing the beauty of the scary situation you find yourself in.

Getting on with it is bravery.

Living with it is bravery.

Dying from it is bravery.

Or, put another way, bravery is finding the courage and the inner strength to try not to blink when the world is telling you that blinking is your only option.

MIDDLE OF THE NIGHT
EMOTIONAL TSUNAMIS

On the whole – in daylight – when I was ill I could tick along pretty well. Relatively speaking, of course. It was at night, though, when my emotions might unexpectedly get the better of me.

I am being strong. I am strong. I am being positive. I am being 'Why Not Me'. I am being cool with it. I am getting on with the day-to-day. I am focusing on other things. I am doing well with the day-to-day. Really well. I get home. I make a tea. The tea tastes like having a mouth full of zinc. But it's fine. It's a reminder. But it's fine. It is fine. I make some food. I don't really fancy food but I need food and I am hungry. But I don't really fancy it. Food. So maybe soup or something? Yes. Soup will be good. Soup will do it. Soup will be fine. And it is. It is fine. It tastes like being force-fed mercury, but it's fine. It's a reminder, but it's fine. It fills a gap. It doesn't quite hit the spot. Well, when I say 'doesn't quite', what I mean is that it doesn't at all hit the spot. But it fills the spot. A spot. So that's fine. Good, almost. I feel a bit light-headed after it but I don't feel as sick as I often do after food, so it's better than almost good. It is good. But even the act of eating/drinking half a bowl of soup has tired me out. And that's a bit weird. I'm an energetic person and a bowl of soup has tired me out. I can't keep my eyes open in front of the telly. But I'm sure that's just tiredness from the day; it's probably nothing to do with the illness. So I can't class that as a reminder. It's fine. Fine. And I'd have been dozing off at this point in the evening anyway. Especially as there's fuck-all on. Except Casualty *and* ER. *And I am up to here with hospitals. So it's more than OK to turn off the telly and have an early night. Maybe a hot bath and an early night. That sounds nice. Sounds normal. My bones being too tired to lift me off the sofa onto my feet isn't normal, though. Is it? Well, maybe it is. Maybe I am just getting old. Maybe even if I wasn't ill, I would be just as completely and utterly exhausted after having got to my feet from a sitting down position. So it's totally normal. And fine. And that hot bath is beckoning me. A hot bath will do it. Will hit the spot. It takes all the effort I can muster to turn on the taps and monitor it to the right temperature but I fill it. I fill it and it's fine. A hot bath always hits the spot. Bubbles. There must be bubbles. I try to get in. I stick a foot in. But it is hot. Maybe too hot. A burst of cold will do it. Just a burst. And it works. And I'm in. But it's a bit cold. It was hot but now it's cold. It's making me shiver and making me feel a bit queasy. It needs some hot. It feels like a bit of a challenge this temperature control thingy and the turning on and off of the taps seems harder than it should be. But the hot goes in. And it's fine. For a moment it's really fine. No, it is too hot. It's too hot. Too hot. And it's making me feel sweaty and wriggly. It's not like the hot bath I had in my imagination. It's not like the relaxing, chill-out, end-of-the-day, 'close my eyes and transport myself to a posh hotel spa' kind of bath that I used to have. I can feel the water scratching my skin. The water is deliberately aggravating me. It's too wet. It doesn't feel like the hot, snug, warm, velvety towel that it used to feel like. It welcomed me in its arms under false pretences. But I guess that's OK. It happens. It doesn't have to be because of the illness. Not every bath has to be beautiful and transporting. I just need to sleep. Just need to rest my eyes, switch off my brain and disappear from the world. And sleep. Tomorrow I will be less tired. Tomorrow I will be less drained. Tomorrow I will be strong enough to face whatever the world throws at me. Although it feels like doing a triathlon, I make it out of the bath, dry off and into the bed. It does feel incredible. Finally being in bed feels fucking incredible. Worth putting up with all that other stuff for. And I am so exhausted that drifting off to sleep without time for a thought or a worry is easy. And immediate. And beautiful. And normal. And normal. And normal. This is one moment of true normality. This little bit now. This first bit of sleep. This bit. The bit where I'm fine. The bit where I don't have to fight. The bit where I don't have to second-guess myself. The bit where I don't have to try and be anything at all. Just normal. And most of the time, that normality, that peace, lasts almost all night. Almost a whole six hours. But this night. Tonight. This night. This night, my tired bones seem to press down hard on my dreams and force me to wake up in a breathless, panicky jolt. And it's instant. The release. It's instant. All that emotional pressure of being the one in control of your illness, being stoic about it, putting everybody else at ease, not thinking about the endgame or at least not thinking that you're thinking about the endgame. All of that stuff that I have unconsciously been holding onto is now pouring out of me in aching excruciatingly painful sobs. Sobs that tear into my soul and feel like my insides being ripped apart bit by bit. Sobs that seem to have no connection or deference to rational thought but that seem to be a giant concoction of blind panic, terror and helplessness. The tears avalanche down my face. My soul demands to be felt sorry for. I fight it at first. Try to get my brain to take over and stop it. But the fighting makes it worse, makes me racked even more, like my bone marrow is bleeding. So I stop fighting it and let it happen. Let it take over me. I throw up my pain but there is nothing left inside me. However, my need gives full force to it and so I retch. I dry-retch until my ribs feel like they have melded together. But the surrendering to it immediately makes it start to dissipate. The surrendering to it makes me able to see the end in sight even as I am doubled over in breathless self-grief. That surrendering allows some rational thought to squeeze its way through my pummelled solar plexus. And as my breathing starts to even-keel itself and I move from the tsunami of sweat that has appeared in the bed, I start to feel both calm and even more exhausted. But calm. And the beauty of what has just happened hits me. I AM normal. I am just ill. For now. And it would be completely and utterly abnormal to sail through this illness and the cunt that is chemotherapy without any physical or emotional lows. Lows that I fight on a daily basis and that my strength and spirit and soul allow me to overcome. In the middle of the night, my body doesn't have the strength or desire to fight any more and it comes out, and it comes out, and it comes out, and however painful that moment is, however upsetting it feels, those are the moments that enable me to make it to the other side of this illness. They are real moments. They are me moments. My moments. They are just as important as the wry, funny moments. If not, more so. So perversely, when they randomly appear, in the midst of the gut-wrenching agony I will learn to enjoy the knowledge that some of the pressure has been taken off. In a strange way I will enjoy the agony because at least I know that I can wake up, the morning after the middle of the night before, to a bit of calm. And I close my eyes and I do sleep till morning and I do feel exhausted from the trauma but I am definitely calm. And it's time for a hot bath. And I need to strip those sheets. The tsunami's over. For now. And the hot bath feels great. And the day begins. And it could well be a good day.*

THE EDGE OF HEAVEN

'Music stops the clock. For three hours, time ceases. It's the one place where for a brief moment you are a master of space and time for real.'

Bruce Springsteen, 2013

Music was my chemo antidote.

It became not only my escape from the darkness but also my escape from the world. Or, to be precise, my escape from the world of reality into the ether of otherness.

Stopping the clock when you have cancer is the order of the day.

EVERYONE NEEDS A BRUCE SPRINGSTEEN WHEN THEY'RE ILL

Bruce Springsteen helped save my life. I have never told him that. I am telling him now. His music opened up the channels of hope to me. It forced me off the floor when I had fallen and couldn't or wouldn't get up. It spoke to me more than any single thing before or since. It shook me and cuddled me and embraced me and told me again and again and again that there was a point to all this. There is a point to it all. Springsteen's music is all about feeling alive and being alive. About finding hope amidst the rubble of reality. Even the most cynical can believe in that hope.

'IS THERE ANYBODY ALIVE OUT THERE TONIGHT?'

Bruce Springsteen in concert is a whole different level of perspicacity and profundity.

It is a spiritual experience.

It is four hours at the gas station of life, replenishing your faith.

The first time I saw him live was thirty-two years ago, front row at the old Wembley Stadium. I was eighteen. I had been a fan of his for about three years. My friend Tort made me a Bruce mix tape (a mix tape that was an actual tape!) when I was fifteen, and the moment I played it, I knew. I knew that this was a game changer. I sort of knew that this was a life changer, too. I didn't quite know yet that this might even be a life saver! Here was a guy who seemed to get me. Here was a guy who seemed to understand my complexities and give full expression to the millions of contradictions going on inside me. Here was a guy who seemed to be able to take my inner turmoil and miraculously turn it into hope and perspective.

I queued for twelve hours to be front row at Wembley, and I looked down on all those people who had just discovered Bruce Springsteen from the *Born in the USA* album. I knew better. I had unearthed my soul to 'Spirit in the Night', shed my boyhood to 'The Promised Land' and planned my escape and world domination to 'Thunder Road'. At eighteen, I made it to the front row.

And the front row felt like a belonging. A small select club.

- The front row to my soul.
- The front row to a religious experience far greater than any eighteen-year-old North London non-believing Jew could ever imagine.
- The front row to a place inside me that, up till then, I was sure didn't exist.

This was pre-YouTube accessibility. Sure, I'd seen a couple of grainy VHS videos. I thought I knew what to expect. I didn't.

It was 4 July 1985.

Something strange happens at an outdoor concert. When that artist walks out on stage he normally does so when it's still light so the thousands of stage lights don't really kick in till later on that night. What you get is this beautiful sepia-like light that never fails to make me want to cry. I don't know why. I am not a nostalgic person but there's something about that light and the wind and the fading sun and the first twangs of music that breaks my stony heart. And I was addicted. I know what addiction feels like and that was it! And it's no use banging on about the Bruce live thing again. Thousands of people have said it will change your life. And it will. It's a direct line to your mind, body and soul. I make no apology for the cliché. For it is as close to a religious experience as I will ever get.

After what seemed like a lifetime of waiting, Bruce Springsteen walked onto the stage alone. One man with a guitar. One ordinary man with a headband. One man who will, in ten years' time, save my life.

He looked up to the skies. They were blue. A blue sky day to lose my Brucinity. Perfect. He looked out to the 80,000 people in front of him. I knew he was looking at only me. He took a performer's moment to take in his world. He didn't say a word and just launched into 'Independence Day'. A beautifully wrought song about the strained relationship between father and son.

And after the fourth line I knew. I knew I wasn't alone. I knew that however scared I was of what my future might bring, I had an equaliser.

And that's the point. **Everybody needs an equaliser**. Some kind of perspective mechanism. Some kind of alkali to all the acid. Bruce live is better than any yogic retreat, better than chanting (though there's a lot of that), better than most sex. He describes it best. It 'rejuvenates'. It's an IV line straight to the soul. More than that. For me, it's a deeply cleansing experience. Washes away the dirt that has collected inside me for days, weeks, years and starts again afresh.

Sadly, the dirt starts to re-accumulate the moment the concert has ended. But that's OK. As any hoarder will tell you, there's something deeply liberating about a life laundry de-clutter.

And going through the ravages of chemo demands constant rejuvenation.

Most days, I wear my game face easily and with a certain amount of pride. I can do this. I can. Get through this. I can. And I do have a surprising and probably innate ability to not let it worry me. Or not let the uncertainty of tomorrow worry me. More than that, I can laugh my way through a lot of it. And about 43 per cent of that laughter is real. I have realised that I am neither a glass half-full kind of guy nor a glass half-empty kind of guy. I am just a guy with a glass kind of guy. Most days I can find enough breath to do much more than just exist. Most days. But chemo is a destroyer like no other. It holds no truck with cocky twenty-eight-year-olds who think they have found the key to indestructibility! And just when you least expect it, it sails on in and lands itself right at the core of your vulnerability and leaves you feeling powerless and weather-beaten and rudderless.

And it was at these moments that Bruce would appear. I wasn't aware of it till years later but he was my ever-present and truest companion on this ride.

- He would show me the right song for the right moment at the right time.
- He would remind me that my immune system might be fucked but my soul was impenetrable.

- He would remind me that fear is impermanent.
- He would remind me that grace in adversity is still grace.
- He would remind me that *searching* for the joy in the now is almost as rewarding as *feeling* the joy of the now.
- He would remind me that without looking deeper into yourself and recognising the darkness that might be there, you can't truly celebrate or even truly recognise the fullness of your humanity.

That's what his songs do and his performances do. They jump from the frothy to the introspective, from the epic to the minute, from the raw to the cheese. To see Bruce live is to celebrate. And to worship. And to think. And to get a bit spiritual. And to cry. And all in all, to have an exhausting but rejuvenating good time. In the nine months that I had cancer I saw Bruce live every single day. I put my fake Discman on (I always had to have the cheap imitation model; it still bothers me), pressed play, closed my eyes and I was there.

And there were thousands of people around me but this one was just for me. And darkness vanished and elation appeared. And hope quickly followed. And life possibilities seemed infinite. And losing wasn't an option. And being alive was an active emotion. A tangible heartbeat thing. And any notion of disappearing was banished. And physical pain was misplaced for just one brief moment. And the tiny flecks of exhilaration at the end of the tunnel grew into a celebration of light, life and being alive. And I was immersed in my very own rock and roll baptism with Bruce as my preacher and my saviour.

Music was my purest means of escape when questions flew around my head that I didn't know how to answer. Music saved me every time I stepped just a little bit too close to the emotional vortex. It stopped me from thinking and allowed me to just live. For that instant at least. To stay alive.

I could write chapter and verse and personal emotional

meaning about most Bruce songs, but I will focus on just one as it's one that gives me life every time I hear it.

'THE PROMISED LAND' BY BRUCE SPRINGSTEEN

'The Promised Land' is an obvious stay-alive song. Obvious but it hits the spot. Stay-alive songs are not about forgetting. They aren't hands over your ears blah blah blah songs. They are the opposite. They are let's face it songs. Let's do it songs. 'The Promised Land' has the most front-foot kick-ass opening of any song past or present. When the harmonica kicks into the drums, your heart explodes, your whole cavity opens up, and at that moment even the most cynical believes.

When I was ill, every time I heard that intro blast into my head, the world seemed to open up into a multitude of possibilities and opportunities. In those eight seconds I knew that it wasn't about living or dying, it was about much more than that. It was about filling and fulfilling every last moment with an unquenchable spirit.

And I can honestly say that twenty-odd years on from that journey, I still get so much strength from those inspirational people who grabbed every single moment and were replete with such grace before death took them. From their strength I must take strength and spirit and soul. From their strength I must learn not to be afraid to smile and to laugh. From their strength I must look beyond the fear of the unknown future and at least try to live absolutely in the moment.

This moment.

This Promised Land moment.

When I was ill, the first step to recognising that I needed to try to rise above feeling shit, both physically and emotionally, was first to accept that a big part of me *did* actually feel like total shit.

Even in the days where I was curled in my bed in the foetal position wanting it all to end, there was a tiny 'fuck you' worm inside me that I knew would eventually take over, force me out of my slumber and out into the world to roar again. Or try to roar. Roaring is good. It feels good. And anybody can do it. Even a mouse can roar!

There were so many times when cancer turned me into an eight-year-old. So many times when the world was giant above me. Kitchen tops were out of reach. Metaphorically speaking, you understand. At five foot eight and a half inches, I am very tall. Very tall. The world felt out of reach. But I would listen to 'The Promised Land' and I would find the strength to rise, take a moment in my hands and feel like me again. Even if only for a second.

There are countless more stay alive Bruce songs, but that's for another chapter in another book. But you get the picture. And my stay-alive songs weren't restricted to Bruce. Hell no. Along the way we had a bit of Oasis, a bit of a Blur and a whole lot of Wham!. Nineteen eighties pop cheese was at the heart of my stay-alive song collection and it was better than any anti-sickness drug or energised pick-me-ups.

I was on the Tube, going to the Royal Marsden for my weekly dose of chemo. I felt light-headed and sick. Not sick enough to actually *be* sick but sick enough to feel nausea 24/7. Which is much worse. The tube is definitely NOT a good place to be when you are in the midst of ball-breaking chemo. I should have taken a taxi. I often did. But when you have cancer *and* a gambling addiction, £13 in a cab is blackjack money, and however close to death you might be, don't fuck with blackjack money. Don't EVER fuck with blackjack money.

I had to be at the Marsden for 10 a.m. to have blood tests to see if my white cell count was high enough to cope with the chemo. If it was too low, it meant that my immune system was too weak to endure the chemo, so the treatment would be cancelled. I was three months in. Side effects were kicking in now. Mouth ulcers, metal mouth, hair loss. Lots of stuff.

Perversely, on chemo day I loved waking up in a ball of sweat feeling like the world or, rather, me was about to end. Why? Because I knew it probably meant that my immune system was fucked and that today would end up being a no chemo day. And that made me happy. It made me relieved. It also made me terrified. It was, as you see, confusing.

So I was on the Tube on the way to the Marsden:

I am dreading chemo today. Totally dreading it. I am light-headed. I feel sick and I just want the entire world to fuck right off. I have this weird thing. I have been doing this chemo thing for a few months now and I have come to know my body pretty well. Apart from the light-headedness and the nausea – which is pretty much constant – I know when my white cell count is down and my immune system low because I get this strange click in the back of my throat. Like something is lodged there that I can't displace. Today is a click day. Today is not a day to be on a crowded Tube. With my immune system this low, proximity is my foe. I am on the Tube, feeling that throat click, knowing I have no immune system, surrounded by commuters. Their every cough, growl or even heavy breath seems to shortcut straight into my soul. I am a juddering, twisting ball of neurosis. Every tiny noise forces me to twist sharply. Away from the coughing bomber. As if to taunt me, to goad me, to pick on me, someone from the direction I have turned to snivels at me at three hundred decibels. It goes on and on and on and I twist and twist and twist. Every time my twist is more defined. More vicious. More ferociously angry. I am the mad guy on the Tube that nobody wants to look at but everybody wants to cough at. I need a badge: 'Cancer on Board. Nobody Breathe!'

It was at times like this that I was desperate for a distraction that would get me away from this human Tube of infection.

A distraction that would circumvent me from this ticking bottomless pit of pain, illness and neurosis.

Wham! is just the remedy.

I hit play on my fake Discman, closed my eyes and got lost in a world of Club Tropicana pop-tastic otherness. And it worked. From King's Cross to South Kensington I was floating on a pop cloud of delirium. Not a cough, a growl or some big man's armpits could get me down.

I *am* at the 'edge of heaven' and I *do* want my 'soul to be forgiven' and I *do* want to get the fuck out of this Tube.

Next stop, South Kensington.

Wham! There is a God.

ESCAPE TO FREEDOM

I am pretty much an insomniac. Never really had an extended period of full, deep and satisfying sleeping. Ever.

There are only two places that I have always slept well:

Hotel rooms and hospital beds.

Hotel rooms have always been the epitome of other. Of fantasy. Of escape. Hospital beds, not so much. They have always come hand in hand with Mogadon or Temazapam. When the nurse came round at 8 p.m. with the pill trolley, I bit the arm that snoozed me. I don't take sleeping pills in normal life but in hospital life I do. And I did. **I so did. Yes**. Please. Prescription sleeping pills not only make you sleep big but they make you dream big. And I am talking 'Lucy in the Sky with Diamonds' big. A legal eight-hour acid trip big.

The only time I have consistently slept well in my own bed was in cancer year. I was drugged up to my eyeballs most of the time, that's why.

STEALTH BOMBING

Having said that, during the second half of radiotherapy, sleep didn't come easily at all. Radiotherapy is much more heinous than chemo. It is the stealth bomber of cancer treatment. Ten minutes of precision zapping, five days a week for three months. That is all. But it takes you on a round trip to hell along the way. Ten minutes of zap. That's all.

You don't feel anything at first. It's fine. The first week and a half are a breeze. But slowly, slowly, it burns into your chest. Physically and metaphorically. **Deeper** and **deeper**.

*Not only is it burning deep into my chest but it is devouring my energy supply until I have nothing left. All my lifeblood, **gone**. Sleep, **gone**.*

And, like I say, sleep was an inestimable commodity. To be treasured like a fragile glass ornament. It wasn't always restful. It was whatever it happened to be that particular night. It was sometimes fitful, sometimes explosive, sometimes upsetting. But it was always sleep and it was always escape. And escape is respite. And respite is priceless.

SPLIT SECOND

Plus, there was always a moment. Always. Without exception. Every time I woke up from a deep sleep. For that split second, I was cancer-free. I was 'normal'. The aliens hadn't landed. No insurgency had taken place. A split second of euphoria fog before the ugly guise of reality descended. Always a split second. And that split second was without doubt the most heartbreakingly magical moment of my cancer life. Every. Single. Time.

This is real. This IS real. This is not a dream. I am clear. I am free. I am cancer-free. I am free of fucking cancer. I am. I am. I do not have stage 4 sclerosing mediastinal non-Hodgkin's lymphoma. I am just me. I have life. I have energy. I am 'me me'. I am ready to get up and go and be the me I remember me to be. In this split second, I am me. Less than a blink of my eye. My split second. All mine. I am cancer free me. YES!

Sadly, that split second of sheer cancer-free euphoria is followed by the biggest crash comedown any addict has ever experienced. Straight in the solar plexus. If I did have any 'why me?' moments, they always came in these spare moments. And this was no split second. This was ten long seconds.

- Ten seconds of self-pity.
- Ten seconds of despair.
- Ten seconds of '*no no no, I can't do this, I can't, I can't do this, I just can't*'.

And then. Peace. My conscious being would take over and check how I was feeling that day.

Do I feel sick at all?

Does my mouth still taste of rusted spoon?

Do I have that weird click in the back of my throat that indicates my cell count is dangerously low?

Am I hungry at all?

Am I ready to face the day?

And once the conscious me took over, I was fine. And in a strange way, that early morning ten-second emotional rollercoaster was my stay alive fuel. Because it felt very real and yet it didn't hang around. It was strong and hard and passionate but it didn't last long enough to wear me out. Just the opposite; it was the gas that allowed me to hit the day running. I wasn't breezing through this thing emotion-free. I had my meltdowns like everybody else but I was blessed with mini bite-sized concentrated ones that spurted inside me and didn't try to overpower my every waking moment.

MY NAME'S RAZ SHAW AND I'M A SMELLAHOLIC

Another useful escape mechanism was smell. If such a person as a smellaholic exists, I definitely am one. I am transported by the good smells and repulsed by the bad ones.

In 1995, lying in a hospital bed, no smell is left unturned! Neither antiseptic. Nor stale sick. Nor mince, potatoes and cabbage. Nor old ladies. Nor death. Nor stale biscuits.

In search of odour neutral, I devour every perfume sample from every magazine in every waiting room of every ward in the entire hospital. I have a giant stash. A dealer-size stash. And at the appropriate moment, I inhale. And I am away, crossing continents, playing backgammon on the beach while drinking bottles of ice-cold Coke, hiking through Andalusian lemon groves, devouring overpriced strawberries while watching a Brit get beaten on an outside court at Wimbledon. For a second, a minute and a moment, the smell takes me out of these sterile confines. The smell takes me to a place called **Elsewhere**.

PARADISE IS A PLACE CALLED ELSEWHERE

Elsewhere is a magical place. A special place. Why? Because it's not **Here**.

It's Elsewhere.

Right now, Here is somewhere you definitely do not want to be. Here is somewhere replete with the unwanted. Here is too real, too much of a reminder, too Here.

I do everything I can possibly do to find Elsewhere. To reach Elsewhere. With my perfume sachet toolkit, I am doing quite well to get away from Here. I am always almost Elsewhere when the overboiled potato fumes of reality plunge me back to the Here. This is prison hell and I am being filthily punished.

HER MAJESTY'S CANCER PRISON

The Royal Marsden Hospital probably has nicer carpets than most prisons. They are a lovely shade of pink. I'm sure the food is better. Sometimes. And as far as I know, my visitors aren't always body-searched before they come in. I told my mum she didn't need to go to such invasive lengths to hide a bunch of grapes and a Dick Francis novel. And it isn't the Marsden's fault. It's an amazing place, amazing facilities, amazing staff, amazing volunteers. Amazing, but it's still a prison. And in prison you are allowed an hour's exercise a day.

In hospital, it's really easy to forget to walk. When your cell count is dangerously low and every tiny movement drains you, staying in bed seems like the only imaginable option. But staying in bed only serves to remind you of where you are. In bed. In a hospital. With cancer. Your will has a daily wrestle with your body and you never know who's going to come out on top. In that particular bout, my resolve is often much stronger and so some walking is done. I say 'some' because I never know how far I am going to get until I don't get there.

I shoe up and ready myself for some real-world walking. Some days I only get as far as the pink carpet in the entrance hall. I *have* to make the pink carpet. That is always my goal. And most of the time, once I've reached the pink carpet it seems sensible to cross the threshold and do the outdoors. Now this isn't exactly encouraged. My cell count is dangerously low and my immune system is shot to fuck. Venturing out into the nonsanitised world that we call life, among real people clearly ridden with God knows what, is a risk of fairly major proportions. But I take the outdoor plunge regardless.

It feels heaven to transgress.

The lifeblood that is pumped into me by this short exterior venture far outweighs any risk that might be involved. I love the utter strangeness of it. I love people looking at me as I wheel my IV drip stand down Fulham Road. With me attached to it, of course. I haven't brought it along to keep me company. My brain isn't that far gone yet.

Of course, if you take that walk too far, you find yourself in hell. And I am not just talking about Chelsea. The body starts to rebel and makes you feel ninety-four again. Most days I know how far to go without going too far but, on the odd occasion that I push it, I pay for it later. My body goes into shock and I am confined to the very bed that I was desperately trying to escape from.

At night-time, I still need to keep this home fantasy going and I make sure I have a tea, a biscuit and something to read at about ten before I devour the pink pills that make me sleep. I am a naked sleeper. Wearing stuff in bed is just weird. Clothes in bed? Clothes are not meant for bed. I have a no-clothes rule when I sleep. Of course, on a hospital ward that becomes a bit tricky. Well, not tricky, so much as dangerous. Not death dangerous but more naked dangerous. If I am going to escape from here at all, I will just have to do it in my birthday suit. There is no other option. Wearing pyjamas in bed in a hospital is so seventies. It's so *Carry on Doctor*. It's so hospital. I couldn't wear pyjamas and escape.

I do actually have pyjamas. I just choose not to wear them in bed.

PYJAMA MANOEUVRES

1.   *Brush my teeth.*

On 350-mouth ulcer days, brushing my teeth feels like scraping the inner cavity of my mouth with a cheese grater.

Instead of a toothbrush, I use a tiny dental floss stick that has absolutely no cleansing effect but does allow me to feel just a tiny bit normal amidst the oral insanity.

2.   *Put my pyjamas on.*

3.   *Take my sleeping pills.*

4.   *Get into bed.*

5.   *After the first wave of drowsiness I take my pyjama top off and put it under my pillow.*

6.   *When the second wave of drowsiness hits, I whip off my bottoms (pyjama bottoms) in a military fashion under the covers, while manically smiling at everyone on the ward to hide my PJ guilt.*

7.   *I leave my bottoms (pyjama bottoms) under the covers within easy reach for re-clothing purposes.*

It works a treat. I am naked under the covers. And naked under the covers makes me feel like normal is here somewhere, watching over me.

Of course, now and again I might forget where I am and get up for a pee in the middle of the night. I often get a few paces away from my bed before I realise that I'm in the raw and have to rush back to retrieve my bottoms (pyjama bottoms).

Naked escape is euphoria, nirvana.

And naked freedom is freedom.

And freedom smells fucking great.

Freedom smells like newly cut grass.

Freedom smells like the fruit/mint mixture in Pimm's.

Freedom smells like Hawaiian Tropic suntan lotion.

Freedom smells like freshly baked bread.

Freedom smells like lemon trees.

Freedom smells like fresh paint.

Freedom smells like petrol.

Freedom smells like shiny new leather.

Freedom smells like woods in rain.

Freedom smells like Playdough.

Freedom smells like the ripping open of a condom packet.

Freedom smells like Grey Flannel aftershave.

Freedom smells like just-popped corn.

Freedom smells like late evening barbecues.

Freedom smells like wet dogs.

Freedom smells like burnt garlic.

Freedom smells like Pepto-Bismol.

Freedom smells like 'other'.

And other is the only place I want to be right now!

IN MEMORIAM?

I know one thing: *life* is to be taken seriously but the moment you take *yourself* too seriously, you are screwed.

However, I can't lie, I don't want stoicism, I want tears. At my funeral. Even more at my memorial service. Bawling, wailing and weeping. European-style, collapsing-on-the-floor lamentation. As a director, I can make that happen. That's the game I'm in. The manipulation game. And in my experience, the best way to make sure people weep uncontrollably is to make them laugh first and then sock them with the sad stuff. They are loosened up and ready to wail!

So you see, I couldn't just die and let someone else plan my memorial service.

ERGO

I am fully aware that a lot of you will wince every time I talk about the possibility of death but it's the reality of that particular situation. The doctor gave me a 70 per cent chance of survival. Ergo there was a 30 per cent chance of me not surviving.

The definition of not surviving is dying.

And, more to the point, those odds give you licence to think about what might happen if you *do* die without actually thinking you *will* die.

The other reason I can talk about it is that I didn't die. You may have noticed. There may well be a Poirot-type twist at the end of this book, but somehow I think that's unlikely.

MEMORIAL

The fact is that I did plan my own memorial service. I couldn't resist it. It was a wonderfully morbid and camp thing to do. And I loved it. That's the point. I had a damn good time doing it. And I didn't do it with 'woe is me' tears streaming down my face. The act of planning my own memorial service felt fun and naughty and liberating. And it was a welcome distraction to the mayhem going on inside me.

DEATH

Plus, the reality of it all is this:

I never thought I would die but I often thought 'what if I did?' and I enjoyed being given guilt-free licence to think such morbid thoughts. A free pass to romanticising my own death. And I devoured it. It was my number one pastime. If you start talking to other people about it, they get uncomfortable because all they see is your death and they find it sad and upsetting that you might be contemplating it. So I chose to keep it to myself.

In truth I found it replenishing. To think about it. To write it down, even. I found glory in going to the edge of the mountaintop. I found glory in the romantic notion of people sobbing uncontrollably at my funeral and again at my memorial service.

DEATH AND THE ELEPHANT

Death and the Elephant creep silently into the room. You can try to ignore the Elephant but you know it's there, squeezed next to your cancer-infested body. Its trunk is playing havoc with your packed lunch. This is the first time that you are faced with the big question. Death.

What do I do? Do I try to ignore it? If I try to ignore it, the elephant rumbles and rumbles and rumbles. And that's not healthy. It's not healthy at all. It's a complete throbbing mind fuck.

Every time you even glance away, its leathery grey skin pushes hard against you and lets out a deep hard trumpeting rumble.

'D-E-A-T-H.'

'D-E-A-T-H.'

'D-E-A-T-H.'

'D-E-A-T-H.'

There's only one thing you can say:

'Elephant (Death), I know you're in here, I know you're close by. I know you could crush me at any moment. But Elephant (Death), I am going to acknowledge you. More than that, Elephant (Death), I am going to get so close to you that I can hear your call. I like knowing you're nearby. I like myself when I know that I am not ignoring you. Not ignoring the possibility of you. That keeps me alert. Keeps me real. Keeps me feeling like I am living in the now rather than running away. It makes Death (Elephant) seem tame or tamed.'

First embrace the darkness. The only way after that is towards the light. The more head-on you can face it, the more you can stare it down, the easier it is to live with and the more likely it is to retreat.

In other words, if we acknowledge death and its potential and possibilities, we are minimising the Elephant and taking the fear of the unknown and the unspoken out of the equation.

It absolutely doesn't mean I thought I was going to die; it purely meant that I could think about death in a slightly abstract and more 'fun' way. Hence the joy to be had in planning my memorial service. That planning made me feel like Richard Burton at Cannes. It is glamour laced with a little bit of darkness. And that's a heady mix. And if Richard Burton is death, then Liz Taylor must be life.

And that's quite a life.

I'll settle for that.

PART THREE: THE RESULTS

THIS MOMENT

This is what all this has been about. This moment. Right now.

The scan.

The blood test.

The prodding and poking.

The looking at the notes.

The looking up at me.

The looking at the notes.

The looking up at me.

It all leads to this moment:

'There's still a mass of something between your lungs but we're pretty sure it's scar tissue and absolutely nothing to worry about. As far as we're concerned, the radiotherapy has done its job and, all things being equal, you're as good as new. We'll see you in three months' time, but, right now, you're good to go.'

And that is that.

I stare straight at her. My consultant. I am full up with silence.

Deafening, fearsome, beautiful, terrifying silence.

That is that.

That

is

That.

I have no words.

Silence.

Silence.

Silence.

I sort of smile.

'Oh! OK. Er. Thanks. OK. Bye then.'

And I am out of her office and into the clinic reception area that I know so well.

I don't want to leave.

What is out there for me beyond these walls?

It's safe in here. It's familiar. I take in what has been my second home for the last nine months. That familiar stale sterile smell. That strange serenity. That calm urgency. Echoes force themselves upon me:

Self-pity tears.

> *Bad cancer gags.*

> > *Strange Wimbledon parties.*

Awkward nurse flirting.

> *Can't find a vein.*

> > *Don't try to speak.*

A Home.

A Home. For. The. Sick

I am homesick.

I find myself in the early spring outside world. A Fulham Road that was always horribly familiar now seems a vast cavern of scary newness that goes on forever.

Nostalgia has never really been my thing. But this new thing, the all-clear thing, the 'you're as good as new' thing, is just plain weird.

Doing cancer is a full-time job. And now I'm out of work.

I spend the next few hours devouring Knightsbridge shops in a sensation void. What should I be feeling?

Euphoric? Relieved? Exhausted? Rejuvenated? Optimistic?

What AM I feeling?

Nothing. I feel nothing. Just dark and numb.

Empty. That's it. Just a big old cancer-free overload of emptiness.

And that's kind of OK. Like this is par for the cancer course. That euphoria or relief or optimism would be tempting fate in some fashion.

So I dismiss it and carry on window shopping.

I say window shopping because, despite having an uncontrollable urge to spend thousands and thousands of pounds on retail therapy, I have an even stronger urge to hit the casino as soon as it opens. So any money spent before that time would be diminishing my gambling destruction stash for later.

And I make it home. To my home. Not hospital home. I make it home with not a penny spilt. And home seems quite different now. Lonelier somehow.

For the last nine months I have been a two-home family and now one of those homes has been taken from me. A huge melancholic wave hits me. Followed by a wave of weirdness. Followed by a colossal wave of guilt. Guilt is my Jewish stalker. It's there at every turn. Every time you think you've banished it, it returns full in the face.

And it is all confusing me.

Why do I feel sad? Why do I feel guilty about feeling sad? Where's the release? Where's the euphoria? I'm an adrenaline junkie. I need euphoria. I need it now. This isn't how I imagined it would be. This isn't what remission is. Remission is supposed to be life-saving, freeing, joyous. Isn't it? This? This is horrible. This is worse than a comedown after a Bruce Springsteen concert.

And then it strikes me what this is. This is grief. I am in mourning.

- *I am in mourning for my ill self.*
- *I am in mourning for the focus that my ill self had.*
- *I am in mourning for the purpose that my ill self had.*
- *I am in mourning for the people who looked after my ill self, for his 'friends' on the wards and in the radiotherapy waiting room.*
- *I am in mourning for my cancer.*

Like two boxers embracing at the end of a mammoth fight, we had squared up to each other and fought a dirty, brutal nine-month bare-knuckle battle. And all I can do as I wave it goodbye is have respect for its power, its resolve and its relentlessness. It has been my opponent, my nemesis, but also my long-term companion. The closest thing to me that I have ever experienced.

And now it is gone. And I miss it. I truly do.

And over the next few weeks that feeling escalated. And as it escalated I went into casino-destroy mode. I reached out for my other powerful opponent and jumped into its dark evil embrace.

And to top all that, after the initial flurry of phone calls when the grapevine learned of my remission, everything went silent.

The phone stopped ringing.

People stopped popping over with food parcels and cheer-you-up gifts. It was silent and I was 'normal' again.

I didn't want to be normal.

Don't turn me back to normal, please. Normal makes me sad and angry and self-destructive.

Casino frenzy intensified.

Something truly horrific began to stir inside me.

Cancer had left me a ticking-bomb-going-home-present-goody-bag.

Inside that goody bag was a note that read:

Please bring my cancer back.

Simple as that.

Every morning I woke up hoping for my cancer to return. Hoping that I could go back to the hell of the previous nine months.

I know that thought is hateful but I had no control over it. Cancer was propped up in the corner laughing at me. It had unearthed my dirty secret. As the guilt deepened, so the gambling frenzy escalated.

The shame was pretty much unbearable.

And it wouldn't go away. It hovered over me like a leopard ready to pounce. And it was confusing. Horrific. Unbearable. It seemingly had absolutely no ending.

Come back, cancer. Please come back. Please, please come back.

My heart imploded in utter confusion. I felt ill and dirty and repulsed. At me. At myself.

Come back, cancer. Please come back. Please, please come back.

And sex didn't help.

Come back, cancer. Please come back. Please, please come back.

And even Bruce Springsteen didn't help.

Come back, cancer. Please come back. Please, please come back.

I tried to talk to other people about it. I tried but it never came out right, and even when it did, they either didn't think I was serious or – much worse – they pitied me and despised me in equal measure.

And the only thing that helped the pain and the guilt was gambling.

CANCER VERSUS GAMBLING, PART FOUR

THE FINAL ROUND

So that's exactly what I did. Gamble. I launched into a pit of utter gambling destruction. Gambling at that moment felt wonderfully horrific. The ultimate in self-harming. Just and deserved punishment for those hateful feelings of cancer grief. And the gambling spiralled out of control. In a matter of just a few weeks I was reduced to maniacal gambling of tumultuous proportions. And I guess the relief that the gambling cult leader felt to have got rid of its cancer rival meant that it was going to grab this opportunity and force me to go completely gambling gaga.

And it did.

And I did.

For me, out-of-control gambling HAD to take place at the casino. Betting shops and fruit machines just didn't cut it. Not 100 per cent sure why. It was something to do with windows. Unlike a betting shop or a fruit machine arcade, a casino has no windows or, at the very least, has blacked-out windows. It has no clocks either. For the simple reason that they want you to lose all sense of time, to get lost in the moment and not think about how long you've been there. So you stay longer. And lose more. A very effective trick that works on addicts and suckers like me. (I am both a sucker and an addict – a saddict.)

I have to emphasise that I didn't KNOW I was out of control. I just knew that I couldn't be anywhere else but the casino at that time. Destruction mode means **not** that you WANT to lose but that you KNOW you are going to. And you don't do anything to stop it. Or, more to the point, you are powerless to stop it! That's the disease. It doesn't allow you the luxury of clarity. It doesn't allow you the luxury of choosing when and where and how you stop being an addict.

Every day for those three weeks I would turn up at Napoleons Casino on the dot of 2 p.m. I'd usually be the first through the door. I loved being first. It was a glimpse of calm before the self-inflicted storm. I went straight to the cashier's desk. How much cash I had was dependent on what had happened on my final bet the previous night. That final bet would often have been at 3.59 a.m. The casino closed at 4 a.m.

It had been nine months since the diagnosis. Nine relentless months of chemo and gambling. It had also been nine months without an income. Unexpectedly, just before my illness, my brothers and I were given £10,000 each after the sale of my grandmother's house. Everyone else seemed to think that this was a lucky financial coincidence that would help support me while I was ill. To me this was gambling money. Pure and simple.

In those three final gambling weeks I got through about £9,000, which was roughly three times the amount of money I actually had left from my original 10k 'stake'. Where I got the rest, I can't even recall. Maxing credit cards? Selling my body? Kidnapping my family? Manipulative lying to the parents? All of the above? Who knows. The fact is that somehow I found the means to fuel the frenzy.

Once inside the casino, blackjack was my game of choice, I would identify a table, nod at the croupier, sit down and begin. In 'normal' gambling mode I would start small – £5/£10 bets – and play conservatively. Warming up, so to speak. However, nothing about this particular mode was in any way 'normal'. This was no time for rational behaviour. It had to be all-out attack from the get-go. Which in play terms meant trying to make twenty-one on almost every hand. This goes against every rule in blackjack strategy school. 'Be patient. Whatever your hand is, you win if the dealer busts'. In destruction mode, you play with £25 chips and you do NOT adhere to the rules. It means you lose big most of the time and win big now and again. Winning big is great. For the simple reason that it affords you more time in the casino and less time in the outside world. Of course, you do EVENTUALLY lose. Need to lose. Have to lose. Want to lose. Do. Lose.

So for those three weeks the gambling beast was unleashed. The gambling cult leader took its revenge good and proper. The self-destruct button was switched to go and I attacked that casino with a furious kamikaze focus that was unlike anything that had gone before or since. And it felt awfully good. And I don't mean that in a Noël Coward way. I mean, it felt fucking awful and fucking good all at once. Like a never-ending vomit to a bulimic. Awful because it *was* awful but good because for the first time in nine months it felt like undisrupted pure focus destruction. And that singularity seemed freedom-like. And freedom was glorious. It was made even more concentrated by a strange feeling in the back of my soul that I couldn't quite pinpoint. A glowing nostalgia feeling. Almost like a final hurrah somehow.

And that's exactly what it proved to be.

10 APRIL 1996

To an alcoholic, their rock bottom is often waking up fully clothed in a pile of their own piss, on a pavement somewhere miles from home. Mine didn't smell quite so bad. At the time, I didn't quite know what triggered the end. But I did know that the contradiction between having been given the all-clear from cancer and then going on a self-destructive gambling rampage was more than crazy and something had to give.

And, with hindsight, there were two significant events leading up to this moment that resonated so strongly within me they must have forced my subconscious to take hold of me, slap me round the face and say, 'Wake up and smell the real world (and the coffee).'

I was in a betting shop. It was what would prove to be the final day of the three-week post-cancer gambling frenzy period. I was gambling on the dogs. I think that first experience when I was twelve years old had convinced me that dog racing was my thing. Not much need to study form or to watch for which dog poos just before the race (the story goes that it makes them lighter so they go faster – a gambler needs every advantage he or she can get!). No. I could smell a winner, poo or no poo.

The truth is that I *was* quite lucky. I could actually pick more winners than losers. Unfortunately, being a gambling addict, my propensity was to bet small money on the winners and big money on the losers. What does that make me? A LOSER!

On this momentous day, I had been in the bookies for about an hour. I had had a few wins. I was up about £500. I was calm. Too calm. I was wary of calm. Calm could lead to thinking and thinking could lead to reality and reality was the very place I was trying to avoid. The reality of the rest of my life. I was not ready for the rest of my life. NOT READY FOR IT. Was still deep in mourning for my cancer.

No, calm must die. Must Kill Calm. Must Destroy Calm.

I know exactly how to do that.

I'll bet all the money I have just won on the next race.

That'll de-calm me.

Definitely.

Now, of course, this was my subconscious speaking and controlling me. The conscious me had no concept of any of this. He just felt the urge to stick all that money on the next bet. And while my subconscious wanted me to lose and thus destroy calm, the conscious me absolutely wanted to win. The bit in the middle, between my conscious and my subconscious (midconscious?), KNEW I was going to lose but wasn't shouting loud enough for me to take any notice of it. Actually, even that's not true. I could hear it but I chose to ignore it.

So with £500 betting slip in hand and race about to start, I stood in front of one of the larger screens in the shop. Next to me was a man who was dressed in a suit and tie that had seen better days. He smelt of a heady mixture of BO and Old Spice. He was probably in his sixties.

The race started. I was on the dog in Trap 2. As it turns out, so was BO-ld Spice guy. Having just relieved himself of any excess excrement (the dog that is, not the man next to me), our dog bolted out of his trap. There was a bump at the first bend and all the other dogs apart from ours and the one in Trap 4 tangled together. That left Trap 2 and Trap 4 neck and neck way out in front. It was one of those races where from a distance it looked like the two dogs were actually one beautiful eight-legged-two-headed beast, so in sync and in stride were they. Such a race is much more adrenaline-raising than if your dog was either winning or losing by a long margin. It's the sort of race that addicts live for. Much like the dogs, me and my Old Spice colleague seemed to be very much in sync, too. Eyes glued to the screen, heads bobbing in time with the dog's stride pattern and in almost choral harmony, a gentle 'go on the 2 dog, go on the 2 dog' escaped from our mouths. The 2 dog slightly pulled his nose in front. Our soft roar turned to full voice now. 'Go on! Go on now!' Coming round the last bend, our dog seemed to have it in the bag; we were preparing our vocal chords for the full-blown dog victory call. A call that's been honed in betting shops and on dog tracks for years and is the musical exhalation of our winning exultation. It goes like this. Are you ready for it? It goes like this:

'OY ,OY,OY,OY,OY,OY, OY, OY.'

This cry is not just a ritualistic adrenaline release but, more importantly, it's a signal to those around you that you're a winner. Or more to the point, that you're NOT a loser. In other words, it's a cry to separate you from your own self-hatred for just a little while.

So.

Final stretch now. We were ahead by half a dog's nostril.

'GWAAAAAAAAN.'

And, just as we were about to give full vent to the victory call, trap 4 took one unfeasibly long, elegant and hateful stride towards the finishing line. Trap 2 was powerless to fight back. Trap 4 literally inched ahead and won the race by a hair's breadth. A dog hair's breadth.

Deflated, defeated and denied my oy, oy, oys, I turned to my neighbour for mutual commiseration. However, BO man had no truck with consolation. He was in his own world of pain. In fact, he was going apoplectic. Bent double, he was ranting and raving in words with no vowels:

'Fkng. Chtng, cnts. Cnts. Cnts. Cnts. Thvng Bstds.'

It was almost as painful to witness as it must have been to live through. And it went on and on and on. I felt pity and disgust for him both at the same time. He was me. I was watching me. It did something to my insides that I couldn't identify but knew was significant. Now I realise what it was. An awakening. Or at the very least, the stirrings of an awakening. I had lost £500 on this race but it seemed irrelevant now. Compared to what he must have lost, emotionally as well as financially. After a few minutes he seemed to have calmed down a touch so I took a moment see if he was OK.

'Bastard dogs,' I muttered

'Ain't that the fucking truth,' he replied

'How much were you on for?' I asked.

'50p,' was his reply. 'My last cunting 50p.'

And that was the moment. The moment I knew. It was game over. For me at least.

Here was a man who was 100 per cent certain that this, his 'last cunting 50p' would not only win him back what he had lost that day but would win him back everything he had ever lost, and some. It would put him back on top.

The point is that:

This. Never. Ever. Ends.

From here on it is just pain upon pain…

It never ends.

So it has to.

END.

HAS TO.

I made my escape. From the bookies, that is.

That afternoon I went round to a friend's house and her brother was there. I was explaining to them both what had happened in the betting shop that morning. Which in itself was a rare occurrence as a gambling addict never talks to any 'normal' people about their losses. My friend's brother then started telling me that he had recently found God (where? I'm not sure. With the 50ps in the back of the sofa?) and that, before finding God, he had been a gambler and a thief. His twenty-four-hour routine in those gambling/thieving days consisted of:

- Identify an easy-to-break-into house (whatever that might be).
- Break into that house at two in the morning and steal 'quick, minor items' such as video recorders.
- At nine the next morning, flog the VCR to someone for twenty or thirty quid.
- Go straight to the bookies and bet that cash till closing time.

Now and again he'd win, in which case he'd have 'a day off the rob' and 'treat' himself to a curry and some weed, but most of the time he'd be skint by mid-afternoon and so would spend the next twelve hours casing up his next house to break into. This cycle went on for about a year until the law caught up with him and he was put in prison. That's where he found God (Oh! That's where God lives.)

It was only on my journey home that I realised how connected the two events of the day were and just how absurd my life had become. I could well end up being either of those guys. What am I saying? I AM either of those guys.

So, the very next day – 10 April 1996 to be precise (I remember the date as it's my brother's birthday) – my body and my soul woke me up, sat me down, looked me straight in the eye and said:

'You're done. Enough.'

And for the first time I listened. For the first time I knew it was over. There was no cold turkey. No huge emotional breakdown. It was over. And it felt pure and brilliant. Pure brilliant. Serenity was my resident now.

I was born again. And it wasn't God I had found. He was stuck in prison. It was a certainty that I hadn't really ever felt before. Put simply, I was certain that I would never again have an urge to gamble.

I knew that I would now be able to walk past a bookies and not feel compelled to go in.

I knew that I wouldn't struggle with it.

I knew I wouldn't relapse.

And more than twenty years on, that is all true. The urge has completely disappeared.

I am a born-again non-gambler.

And in all the research I have done since, that is very unusual. The gambling addiction world mirrors that of any other addiction. It is littered with relapses and worse. So I don't know how I got out of it so sharply and cleanly. I guess those heavy-duty chemo drugs ended up killing everything that dared to get in their way.

Chemo cult leader? **Dead.**

Gambling cult leader? **Dead.**

No pains in my chest.

No deep-seated desires to be ill again.

No urges to self-destroy.

No urges to gamble.

Just calm.

I had found my promised land. For a moment at least. The struggle to the mountaintop was vicious. I didn't know when or where or *if* the zenith would come. But it did. Come. And it was serenity itself at the top. And today I can at last look forward to tomorrow.

I had destroyed such a huge gaping hole in my wall of pain that, in the end, it was easier just to walk through it and leave it behind.

All I could do was hope I would come out the other side alive.

And I did. I have.

And I haven't gambled since. And I have been cancer-free since.

Don't get me wrong. I have had numerous moments of self-destruction since. Of course I have. But they have been both much less extensive and much more isolated. Plus they were never to do with gambling but were almost always connected to sex in some fashion or other.

I can still feel that cancer-wish fulfilment lurking somewhere inside me. It's an evil, poisonous monster. Like grief, I know it won't go away completely. It rears its head at the most unexpected times. The difference now is that not only is it much easier and quicker to banish, but I can now go ages without feeling guilty about it.

Only ages, mind. Not never. Like I say, guilt is in my DNA.

And I have come to understand that the stabbing desire for cancer to return is a really common feeling. Better the devil you know and all that. And once someone has been given the all-clear, to have that feeling pop up to surprise them not only shocks them but it also fills them with self-hatred.

Seeing a friend breathe out a little bit when I explain to them that they are not alone in having those feelings is a privilege that I can't explain in words. It's the privilege bestowed on me by the cancer club. And sometimes someone telling you that you are not alone is useful and comforting and other times it doesn't help one jot.

But my experiences might resonate at some point, when you're ready to take them in, so it feels right to put them out there.

And though I have never really subscribed to the notion of cancer bringing me a whole new positive perspective on life, I can definitely say it brought me to a place of some clarity. I had to wade through Dickensian smog to get there but I did find some.

And now, when the haze of irrational madness descends – and it does descend fairly regularly – I step into it for a while just to remind myself how hateful and all-consuming it feels. And I know it will pass. And I know it will always be a part of me.

Clarity comes and goes. Perspective comes and goes. But some memories get drilled into your mind more deeply than your consciousness and, even when you think you've forgotten them, they are always there. Manipulating your decision making.

Here are some things I know:

- Those three crazy post-remission self-destruction weeks in hell were the kick-start to the person I am now.
- Those three crazy post-remission self-destruction weeks in hell sit in my skull as a reminder of a world I never want to return to.
- Without feeling the full throttle of those three crazy post-remission self-destruction weeks in hell, I would never have escaped it.

So, you see, cancer ended up a giver more than a taker.

Cancer gave me a new focus.

Cancer gave me a wake-up call.

Cancer gave me an empathy, an understanding, and an ability to help others.

Cancer gave me my life back.

Dear 28,

As a twenty-eight-year-old, I didn't know whether fifty was going to exist for me or not. I thought I might get to see twenty-nine, but even then I wasn't certain. In essence it wasn't that I didn't think that I wouldn't die, more that I couldn't imagine NOT being around for another year. If that makes any sense (double negative madness). And it was that little bit of uncertainty that gave me fuel to make sure that my motor did more than just tick along.

I am glad this letter won't actually reach you, because I don't really want to tinker with that motor. It's a big reason that I am still here.

Besides, going back to the future is so eighties!

When I was you, I had to keep reminding myself that 'future' wasn't a dirty word. That thirty, thirty-five, forty-five or even fifty might be a realistic proposition. Not a dream, or a fairy tale. And that 'now' was the greatest word of the lot. My 'now' was twenty-two years ago. And now. Twenty-two years feels like a lifetime ago. And yesterday. I always told myself then to trust in my instinct. I wasn't totally sure that was true back then. Now I'm sure. How do I know I'm sure? Easy. Instinct!

Why am I writing to you in this slightly self-conscious way?

I have an instinct that reconnecting to my twenty-eight-year-old self will be really useful to the fifty-year-old me. I haven't quite worked out why yet. Or even how. I may discover it along the way. I guess a big part of me is wondering if I have turned out the way you might have imagined I might.

Was all that fight worthwhile?

I think the reason it took twenty-two years to write this book, and indeed to properly communicate with you, was that I was always scared that the answer to that question might actually be NO.

That I wasn't worth fighting for.

That I might be a disappointment to twenty-eight-year-old me.

That nothing was gained by my survival.

And I guess the reason that I have faced this now is that it has taken me twenty-two years to come to a still slightly hesitant, positive response to that question.

As a twenty-eight-year-old, you burnt inside with the need to ask for help but you had too much pride to admit to the world that you needed that help. For the next few years, despite surviving a life-threatening illness, things didn't really change. However desperate you might have been to reach out to someone, your own contrary antagonism forbade it. And that was so boring and painful for everyone. Especially you.

I am now an ancient man of fifty and thankfully, finally, the walls of belligerence might be starting to crumble and an antidote to the fierceness might be in sight. I see a life worth living and a life worth being saved for. I see a perspective worth writing about. Life IS weird and perspective is our biggest crutch. We forget so quickly and then feel guilty for forgetting. We shouldn't feel guilty. We should just keep re-remembering.

Twenty-eight, if you could read this, the biggest thing I would want to say to you is this:

Along the path of the next twenty years, take pause to breathe and try to accept help when offered. And even when you can't, which is most of the time I suspect, be gracious in your refusal.

I need you to know that I have thought of you every day for the last two decades. You have made me what I am becoming today and I will always be grateful for that.

I owe my life to you.

Yours always.

50

EPILOGUE

In my nine-month fight to the finish, I came out ahead. Just.

There were moments along the journey where cancer pulled away so far that I thought I'd never catch up, and other times where I went into cruise control thinking I had it licked, only to find it overtaking me on the inside rail.

It was only once it was all over that I really looked back at the race and realised how close it had been. And it was only then, as now, that I was able to think about and honour those who didn't make it.

Tiny margins. That really is all it is.

And in this race, it's not skill or hard work that leads you over the finish line in front. It's circumstance. And luck. And that's the terrifying and heartbreaking thing. All this is pretty much out of our control.

THE BODY HAS THE LAST WORD

We can manipulate the way we choose to live our lives at this time. We can even determine who we want to spend it with and how. We can manufacture an environment that makes life as bearable as possible. But we can't determine whether we live or we die. Even the best oncologists in the world can't determine that. They can do as much as they can do. And that's a lot. But ultimately it's the body that has the last word. It's the body that is more powerful than anything else. It's the body that determines the why and how and if. We have no control. We are left feeling like we are treading water in quicksand without a life jacket.

MINIMISE THE WHOOPING

That's why it's hard for me to say that living with cancer and surviving makes me appreciate life more. So much is governed by fate. So much is out of my jurisdiction. So much is about good or bad luck. The finest way we can honour those who didn't make it is just to get on with our lives without too much whooping and hollering.

He says, having just written a book about it!

It would be a lie to suggest that living when I could have easily died has not made an impression on my life. Of course it has. But I don't skip around town, loving everyone and everything, shouting, '*Woo, I love life. I so love life.*' Just the opposite, in fact. I am less tolerant of things or people that seem to waste my time. Because the clock is always ticking.

PERSPECTIVE

The realisation that it's a very thin line between existing and not existing *does* offer you perspective. I say 'offer' because it is so easy not to accept it. Or, more to the point, it is easy to forget that it's there. But it *is* there, with a positive stealth-like life of its own. In the midst of a moment of overblown stress, perspective will appear and insist on you calming the fuck down. And that's a bonus and a blessing.

It affects every part of my life, especially my work. It's the reason that most of the time when there's a crisis, I find calm. Ice calm. There's no point in getting too worked up about stuff. That's really not going to help. Anybody. When I look back at my twenty-eight-year-old self, I see a boy trying to be a man wanting to be a boy. At fifty, I am learning to be comfortable in the skin that I am in. I am learning. I am close. There is no cigar.

BRUSHING SHOULDERS WITH DEATH

In nine months I became more intimate with death than I might ever have imagined. I not only brushed shoulders with it, I shared a bed with it, wrestled naked with it and exchanged bodily fluids with it. I might not like it, it might not be my friend, but I am very comfortable with it. I am not lost for words in its presence. I am not in awe of it. I have debilitated its power and allowed myself the luxury of living without fear of it. And that not only gives me the confidence to take risks where previously I might have been more cautious, but it also affords me insight that can be used to help others.

POST-CANCER BANDITS

Death, however, does like to remind you of its presence now and again, just in case you get too blasé about the whole thing.

I was in Mexico City about four months after having been given the all-clear. I was in full post-cancer recuperation mode. I had been there for a few weeks staying with friends when some other friends came out for their summer holidays. We all decided to take a trip to see the Pyramids of Teotihuacan, just outside Mexico City. We got a bus there. Had a rather lovely time. At the end of the day, got a bus back. Six of us and eight other tourists.

The journey from Teotihuacan back to Mexico City is quite a straightforward one. In fact, that's exactly what it is. Straight and forward on an A road/Mexican motorway-type thing. It was fiercely hot. The bus was old and lacking many things. Including air conditioning. Along the way, there were a number of stops. They didn't seem to be official bus stops. The bus just stopped. About twenty minutes into the sweaty journey, the bus made one of those impromptu stops and five people got on. They all seemed to know each other. Four men and one woman.

I noticed that they didn't all sit together. Odd. Another ten minutes went by and one of them stood up quite sharply. It was all a bit of a snapshot blur after that. A man stood in front of me brandishing a toy gun. I say 'toy' because that was exactly my first thought: *'These Mexicans, they have a strange sense of humour.'* I interrupted that thought with an ice-cold realisation that this was no toy. The five of them were spread around the bus, systematically ridding everyone of all their possessions. There was screaming, and guns to heads, and sweat. Lots of sweat.

A man with a comically large moustache calmly, and with half a smile, put a gun to my head and beckoned me to give him all my stuff. I gave him my wallet and he took the cash. He took my camera. I didn't want him to have my camera. It had pictures of my trip, and despite my lack of nostalgia, pictures of this trip represented something. They represented the now. They represented recovery and, more importantly, they represented the beginning of tomorrow. So I pleaded for it and amazingly he dropped the gun from my head and gave it back to me. The camera, that is. Not the gun. I think I was so shocked by the fact that he was actually giving me my camera back that I was all fingers and thumbs and accidentally pressed the shutter release and the flash went off. Oops! There was lots of shouting from all around the bus. The gun returned to my head and moustache man grabbed the camera from my hands. At that moment I genuinely thought he might pull the trigger.

Eventually the banditos got off the bus and ran into the fields. They disappeared through the long grass like a Mexican *Field of Dreams*. We stopped at a motorway police station. The police – clearly bored – rounded up ten police cars and two helicopters and managed to capture them all almost immediately. They brought them back to the police station while we were all still there and, much to our liberal confusion, they beat them to a pulp in the back room. We could hear every blow. We spent the next eleven hours in a one fan/one typewriter police station, giving endless sweaty statements.

And that night I had a meltdown.

It was due.

I had been sailing through this trip, sailing through my recuperation, not really stopping to think about all that had happened over the last year.

Then some amateur bandits got on a bus.

The irony hit me hard between my gringo eyes. I had exhausted so much energy in my cancer sparring match only to be killed by a rusty gun on an old bus by a sweaty, stale-smelling, terrified Mexican on a rickety road back to Mexico City. Bueno!

The ridiculousness of that notion seemed to strike right at the heart of me. I realised, almost for the first time, just how close to death cancer had taken me and quite how seismic the last nine months had been. It was only at that moment that I understood quite how much effect the events of the previous year had had on the person who came through the other side.

At that moment, fear and pain and anger and pride and buckets full of relief poured out of me. At that moment I realised what the biggest lesson of this whole cancer experience was going to be. And it was this.

THIN LINE

You can only truly taste life if you accept that there's a thin line between pain and pleasure, love and hate, and, yes, life and death. If we expect just to feel empty of darkness because we have survived a life-threatening illness, then we are going to spend the rest of our lives chasing something that can't be reached. The elephant is always a mere trunk's length away.

Cancer taught me that it's OK not to be happy all the time if I can allow the possibility of being happy some of the time. In other words, I have given myself a guilt-free pass to be grumpy. Perfect.

Cancer has taught me that there are always smiles to be found, however dark the situation. Those smiles are always restorative, even for just one moment. One moment of joy can loiter and linger much longer than you might ever have imagined. One moment of joy can help you deal with the hideousness in front of you because it doesn't just exist in the now. It exists as a resonating memory to draw on whenever you most need it. A tiny steam spurt in the pressure cooker of cancer. Tiny maybe, but a much needed release nonetheless.

HIGHS AND LOWS

Having said that, people often question why I never seem to get overexcited about anything. Except a Bruce Springsteen concert on a balmy summer's night, of course. It is absolutely the product of this whole experience. BC, I was the addiction adrenaline king. And I would demonstrably express life's peaks and troughs. But that was before perspective came into my life.

Perspective is like a good wine. It deepens with age. It is an open gateway to calm. And calm *is* the promised land. Calm feels like respect for those around you. Calm feels like a realistic appraisal of the truth of the situation as opposed to a made-up reality seen through self-obsessed eyes. Calm feels like the thing to chase. Not highs and lows. I have trained myself not to get lost in over-exuberant highs. They are both egotistical and risky. The higher the high, the more painful the crash. An over-indulged high can be the beginnings of losing that perspective that I have nurtured and cherished for so long. And calm feels achievable.

Do I always realise that calm? Hell, no.

Was I calm when a bandit held a gun to my head? Externally

maybe, but my still skinny arse almost pooping itself might have been a bit of a giveaway. Besides, a little bit of fear is a good thing.

Walking through a door to a new world, tackling something you don't completely understand or dealing with people who are relying on you can be petrifying. That fear feels paralysing to start with but then it becomes the fuel to spur you on, move you forward and deal with whatever the thing is. Fear keeps you real and keeps you alert.

Surviving a life-threatening illness doesn't make fear disappear. It just takes the edge off its power and affords you the insight, clarity and courage to walk into it rather than run away from it.

THE CANCER ROAD

Everybody has their moment. It comes at different times in different ways for different people. Even though I always wanted to be a wunderkind, cancer made me realise that it's never too late to make your mark.

And that's why, if I had my time again and I was given the choice, I would absolutely take the cancer road. The other one is calmer, less bumpy and nowhere near as challenging. But I am learning that I need a challenge. That is the way I win. That is the way I make my mark.

Challenging cancer has also blessed me with clarity. The self-same clarity I thought I didn't possess as a frustrated twelve-year-old. Clarity to see straight to the emotional heart of a situation. Clarity to find the right words for the right person at the right time. Clarity to jump into a difficult situation rather than shy away from it. I don't always succeed but the act of trying is often just as powerful.

Cancer was not only the biggest challenge; it was also the

greatest teacher. It educated me not only about human emotions but also about humanity itself. It allowed me to engage with feelings I might have otherwise buried, and encouraged me to try to see the world through other people's eyes. It taught me that self-obsession is much more harmful than any cell-eating disease and that one word of useful advice to someone else is worth a thousand first places and ten thousand winner's trophies. I didn't really know any of this three years ago. It was only in the act of writing this book that I made these discoveries. Prior to this, they had lain dormant in the dusty cellar that is my soul for years.

TRIPLE-COOKED CANCER CHIPS

After all, I'm a would-be spiritual person. A spiritual wannabe if you like. And a cynic. I am not sure that the two are not mutually exclusive. The older I get, the less cynical I want to be and the more I am trying to embrace my experiences rather than run away from them. Which is why I am writing this book now and not fifteen years ago.

For a long time, I had a big old cancer chip on my shoulder. I can't really define how that manifested itself, but I know it was there. I could almost smell the Sarson's vinegar. To other people and often to myself, I was really upfront about my cancer experiences. I appeared honest and open. I loved being told that my story was a remarkable one. I loved shooing away the '*you've been so brave*' comments as if it was water off a duck's back. The truth, of course, was that comments like that puffed me up. They validated me. They were my new drug of choice. And it was all just a bit of a façade. It was a great mask to hide behind. The honesty mask. The bravery mask. The '*he's dealt with it so well he can even make inappropriate jokes about it*' mask.

What was the mask really hiding? I am no guru when it

comes to myself, but, in very simple terms, the mask was a shield to stop me having to deal properly with stuff. The 'honest and open' me was a brilliantly manipulative way of fooling everyone, including myself, that I was embracing the future without ignoring the past.

Only now am I realising that my cancer was a much bigger deal than I allowed myself to perceive at the time. I have lived in its shadow for years. It had been haunting me, in fact. I was the fifteen-year-old again who – ferociously searching for a unique identity of his own – walked into a theatre and found a home.

Cancer had become my master. My unpredictable master. My safety blanket, too. My mask. Whenever I needed to make myself feel unique I would reel out the cancer story, and people would inevitably sit forward and listen. And for a moment I would feel special and different and free. But I also felt cheap. This is all hindsight, you understand. At the time I wasn't aware of bringing out the cancer card and I didn't really equate feeling a bit shit with all this. This had become my Unique Selling Point if you like. It had become so much a part of me that I couldn't see the join.

And, looking at it now, I buried my personality inside my cancer story. Because that was a comfortable place to be. A place I understood. A place where my innate shyness disappeared and I had a captive audience. A place where I seemed to be what I always wanted to be:

Winning and Unique.

And it's only really been in the process of writing this book that I have realised the extent to which I submerged my own self into my cancer self. The extent to which I had truly hidden. I am good at hiding because I hide in a very loud, abrasive, larger than life public way. While people are seeing me one way, the real me is usually cowering behind that giant-sized mask. And it's draining. More than that, it's unsettling both to me and to whoever I am with. And even beyond that, it never allowed me to be truly one strong, focused individual.

The more I talked about my cancer, the more I was able to convince myself that I had dealt with it. With the enormity of it. When I came to write a book about it, I realised I hadn't. I really hadn't. All that free and easy talk was just that, really. Free and easy. It hadn't penetrated the surface at all. And then something changed.

SURPRISED BY YOUR OWN STRENGTH

It changed when a close friend of mine had the honesty and courage to share with me the pain and fears about the cancer of her mother. These conversations normally took place while watching Arsenal. A pain of a different kind. My friend's honesty was so moving to me, so beautiful, that it changed my life. It made me realise that if I could help her just a little bit, even if only for one moment, then it will all have been worth it. And by helping her, by helping Jo – I'll call her Jo as that's her name – I was also helping myself because after eighteen or so years there was a lot of my own stuff that I had conveniently buried. Jo's honesty and her mum's determination to find joy amidst the pain and the suffering was incredibly inspiring to me. That inspiration springs from an awareness of how much effort it takes to not cave in to the pain, both physical and emotional, that you encounter daily when dealing with a life-threatening illness. It's the surprise of your own strength and spirit that I'm really fascinated by. A spirit that you almost definitely don't know is there until you are forced to search for it. And it's that very spirit from Jo, her mum and countless others that inspired me to revisit my twenty-eight-year-old self and write some of my thoughts and feelings down.

And I pretty much found my identity again when I started helping others deal with their pain and forgot about my own.

Almost by osmosis my numerous selves began to merge. And a new, calmer, more singular me began to appear. And for almost the first time, I was in control of myself and of the perception of myself that I was able to give to others. And, seven years on, I find that I quite like myself. Quite. I don't need to hide behind cancer to have a large personality. Just the opposite, in fact.

I am still the inappropriate, sometimes loud, often needing to be centre of attention guy that I always was. More so, even. And I like that side of me. It makes me smile that I can be like that. I just have much more of an ability these days to control it when the time is right.

And the writing of this book has made me understand that change in a much more conscious way. It has made me appreciate the now that is today. It has allowed me to express the larger side of my personality more than I might have ever felt comfortable doing. And it has made me more able to step away from my cancer story without the fear that I might lose myself in the process. (Apart from writing this book, of course – contradictions, contradictions, contradictions!)

It has made me realise that the darkness of looking into the face of death and embracing what's there or what's not there is the very thing that reawakened the lightness in my soul.

I can't describe it any other way. Finding the beauty in this hideous illness is hard, sometimes impossible. But beauty comes in many forms.

Clarity is beauty.

Insight is beauty.

Generosity is beauty.

Forgiveness is beauty.

Acceptance is beauty.

Fear without bitterness is beauty.

Discovering that soft, sweet-smelling baby hair is growing back on your misshapen bald head is beauty.

Above all, the writing of this book has made me realise that it's absolutely not about first place or second place, it's about finding the right place.

And if that ain't just a little bit spiritual, fuck knows what is!

APPENDIX 1

Below is a short play that was commissioned by Paines Plough – a touring theatre company specialising in new writing and new work – for a show that was known as Directors' Perform. The premise was that they would pair up a director and a writer who'd worked together a number of times, and the writer would write a short monologue for the director to perform. Presumably so the writer could get their own back for the number of times that director has asked the writer to butcher/delete/rewrite some of their precious script. I have worked a lot with the brilliant Naomi Wallace, and she wanted to write something about my cancer, my gambling addiction and my love for Bruce Springsteen. Naomi has kindly agreed for it to be shared with you here. I did indeed perform it, for one night only, at the Soho Theatre some years ago. No live record of it exists. Thankfully!

WORD'S A SLAVE BY NAOMI WALLACE
(DEVISED FROM CONVERSATIONS WITH RAZ SHAW)

(The stage is bare. After some moments a man in his late thirties/ early forties appears on stage, dressed casually. He eyes the public.)

I did three things when I got ill. Gamble. Chemo. And listen to Bruce. And not necessarily in that order.

Shakespeare knew exactly what I'm talking about:

'I have seen a medicine
That's able to breathe life into stone,
Quicken a rock, and make you dance canary.'

And baby, once you dance the canary, no other dance will do.

Our second Bard, Bruce Springsteen, knew this too.

(He sings a couple of lines from the Bruce Springsteen song 'Growing Up'.)

So here I am, holding my breath and dancing the canary, dealing the medicine of the blackjack God to my right and to my left, and turning my skin over and over and inside out again and again and I'm losing and I'm losing and I'm losing but then I'm winning and I'm winning and I'm losing again, I'm losing again, I will not get up from this table, I will not get up from this cunting table because it feels too good and I can win again and it feels too good and I will win again...

And then it's silent. The canary stops singing.

Sure it can kill you. The gambling. The cancer too. But then there's almost nothing in this world that won't. Kill you. But before it does, it'll flash your blood and send a sting of heat 'cross your gums, down your throat and into your gut. It's a kind of sustenance.

I've always maintained that I don't gamble, I pray. And I practise this form of prayer sitting down, standing up, or crawling on all fours. And once I get to praying, there is a continuous flow of time 'cause time changes its dimension when you twist and stick. Time no longer passes, it just quits. And because it quits, it can't take you with it so you just stay. Still: pure focus. I sat in Atlantic City for twenty-three hours straight at a blackjack table, taking only a few, quick shifts to piss, shit, drink water from the bathroom sink and eat handfuls of salted peanuts. I didn't wash. Didn't brush my teeth. But in those hours I felt more pristine, more vigorous, more perfected than I had in my entire life.

(He sings a line from the Bruce Springsteen song 'Born to Run'.)

Ace. An Ace from God: right here.

(Thumps his chest once to show location.)

Top of my chest between my lungs.

Yeah, folks don't say it but I see it in their flat little faces: I was at the height of my gambling when I got sick. Was God punishing me? Was cancer my private message from God? My answer: Would it matter? Would it really fucking matter?

What mattered was that one day I went T.F.B. Street tag: Totally Fucking Bald. Six months chemo and I mean no hair anywhere. Neither sprout nor sprig to be found in crack or fold. And then I began to swell. From all the steroids. And it was like taking an air pump on full power to a garden variety worm. The contours of my body just stopped guarding their borders. Then came the side effects, 350 of them to be exact, and all at one time: mouth ulcers. So for a while there I couldn't speak and I couldn't eat. Let's say I was not at my most devilishly attractive.

But that didn't stop me from attending my personal synagogue. I kept going back, with my hairless head, to that place of smack-against-the-table, 'Card, Please.' Blackjack.

'Course it's a form of escape. A kid could tell you that, but for all the places I've sat down in my life, it's the only one that truly feels like home.

It was the same with Bruce. You see, The Boss might not be the greatest musician that ever lived and his voice, well, between him and me, sometimes I think my croak is more muscular than his. But the package that is Springsteen is a heat-seeking device that won't rest till it tracks you down, locks on hard and slaps you spinning till:

(He sings a line from the Bruce Springsteen song 'Badlands'.)

Whenever you're fucked in your head or your gut or your groin, Bruce is like your own personal toolbox. Trite, sure. But that doesn't make it less real. As were the needs of my system when I sat down at that table and was repeatedly flushed, irrigated with a liquid God: epinephrine.

Street tag: Adrenaline. Nectar from the adrenal glands when danger threatens, hence the rush. Yeah, the rush. It's a cliché that we gamble for the rush. But a rush is not just a hit or a high. It's total body dominance: hard, sharp and thorough.

Ace: Stage 4 sclerosing mediastinal non-Hodgkin's lymphoma of the large cell type.

Street tag: Cancer of the lymph you're-fucking-dying glands. And you Can't Walk Away. Under. Any Circumstances.

(He sings a line from the Bruce Springsteen song 'I'm on Fire'.)

Some say there's a bigger rush in losing than there is in winning:

Stick 'em up. Your money or your life. Sure. And yet there were times when I was so scared my teeth hurt.

There is a kind of kick-ass arrogance about being a part of the cancer club. You no longer say to women, 'Haven't I seen you somewhere before?' A simple 'I got cancer', occasionally followed by 'baby', gives you more mileage than a wallet full of cash. It's a status thing. I mean, whatever your natural standing might have been before you got sick, cancer shoots you to the front of the line. People who made you feel small now seem tiny to your bigness. Therefore, I developed T.C.S. Street tag: The Cancer Swagger. Translated simply as 'I don't roll the dice, I AM the dice.' So during my illness I actually got quite a lot of what I saw as freakish sympathy sex and I'd be lying on my back, in all my bald glory, with some shit hot chick shaking roulette on top of me and thinking: 'Baby, are you mad!? I look like a fucking alien.'

But I'd wipe myself off and head back to my church where I'm losing and I'm still fucking losing and...

(He sings a line from the Bruce Springsteen song 'Backstreets'.)

... and I'm losing and I'm losing but then I'm winning and I'm winning and I'm winning and I'm winning and I'm losing, I'm losing, I will not get up from this table, *(he hums)*, I will not get up from this table, *(he hums)*, I will not get up from this table, *(he hums)*, because it feels too good and I can win again, it feels too good, *(he hums)*, I will win again.

And then on a day like any other day it goes silent. The canary stops singing.

And God sits down at my table and smiles at me.

I'm not that surprised; I've been praying to him for months now, days, hours, and I never let up.

(He sings a line from the Bruce Springsteen song 'Brilliant Disguise'.)

So God shows me his teeth 'cause he's proud of me. And suddenly I'm no longer alone. I stink and I'm hungry and I'm tired and I'm broke but I'm ready to deal again. Always ready to deal again. But when God smiles at me I see he's got something stuck in his teeth. It's small and green and nasty. But I'm fascinated. I'm hooked.

I put down my cards, just for a second, and move in close 'cause I got to see what God's got trapped in this one spot between his canines, and as I get closer I smell God's breath and it's so sweet, so dark that I want to crawl inside and stay there.

But then I see what it is, caught like a piece of last night's dinner.

It's me. That piece of flotsam between God's teeth is me. And before I can even let out a whimper, God shoots me a card. All right, I say. Let's play. I turn the card over. Bingo. Alleluia. Oy-fucking-vey.

And while I can't read the card, which reads like a smear down a window, I know what it means: **I am not going to die.** Jackpot. Pretty penny. Windfall. The cancer in my lymphs will soon be packing its bags, heading on down the road to torment some other loser.

So for now, I've been given the green light to fuck the hell out of gambling as I'm about to wave goodbye to both the cancer and cards and the madness forever. Soon, yeah, real soon.

(He sings three or four lines from the Bruce Springsteen song 'Badlands'.)

The first time I entered the casino in remission, I missed my sidekick, my non-hodge-lymph. Sure, I was glad it was walking away, though I was colder somehow.

But hey, today it's still an ace. Deal it. Fuckin' deal it. Over and over and over till I'm emptied and so absolutely still inside I can't remember what fruit tastes like, what water feels like on my arms, how quiet and thick the night can be when you just fall easily asleep.

Soon, yeah, real soon.

But no matter how hard I play and stay and pray, God's never sat down at my table again.

(He looks for a moment at the public, and then exits.)

The end.

APPENDIX 2

Excerpt from *Gambling* by Tom Holloway, a play devised by me and co-directed by me and Georgina Lamb about my gambling addiction.

It was produced by Eleanor Lloyd and performed at the Soho Theatre in 2010.

I walk along the row of machines until I find the one that
    feels right.
That's my ritual.
To find the machine that's talking to me.
Calling me.
I walk along and then I find it.
It looks like all the others.
It sits there just like all the others.
But this is the one for me today.
Today we will go on a journey together.
Today it is my partner.
I sit down in front of it on the little black stool.
It swivels just right.
Everything feels just right.
I put my money down.
My little cup of money.
I keep my handbag in my lap as I sit down and put my little cup
    of money down in front of me.
I love the cup of money.
The cup of coins.
Heavy.

I love how heavy it is.

Waiting for me.

A whole cup there just waiting for me.

The machine.

The stool.

The cup.

Everything is ready.

Everything is right.

This is the moment I love.

The screen glows in front of me.

One of the local girls places a complimentary glass of lemonade in front of me.

She smiles at me and gives me my drink and says it's lovely to see me again.

She uses my first name.

Her.

The machine.

The stool.

The cup.

All of it inviting me.

All of it welcoming me.

This is the moment I love.

This is where it feels good.

I reach in to the cup.

I take out ten coins.

I slide them in to the machine and it comes to life.

Here we go.

You and me.

It talks back.

Sings its little songs.

Invites me to press its buttons.

Inviting me in to its game.

I love the first press of the button.

I feel it…
I feel it deep inside me.
I move my hand up.
Place my finger right on the glowing button and I…
I…
I…
push.
I place just one finger on it and I push and we have begun.

I get small wins.
To begin with.
Five credits.
Seven credits.
It's teasing me.
I enjoy it.
Just when I'm almost out…
Five more credits.
Ten more credits.
I watch the shapes spin on the screen.
Each time.
Game after game.
Spinning there in front of me.
Sometimes flashing.
Sometimes it sings.
But always spinning.
Every game spinning.
I up the ante.
I'm enjoying this.
I up the bet.
It asks for more money.
I oblige.
It's teasing me and I'm saying to it, tease me more.
Reel me in.

Do your worst to me.
Push the button.
The images spin.
Push the button.
The images spin.
I hear someone.
Suddenly I hear someone on another machine.
Lights and sounds.
A big win.
Five hundred credits.
I know it just by the sounds of the machine.
Five hundred credits.
They're working together now, these machines.
Dancing with me.
Toying with me.
And I love it.
Bring it on.
You lead and I'll follow.
I push the button.
I follow you around the room.
I push the button.
We move with grace and poise.
I push the button.
Lights up.
Your song plays.
One hundred credits.
Showing me I can do it too.
Giving me a little taste of the big win I just heard.
Seeing my cup is almost empty it gives me a nice win to keep
    my game going.
This dance.
This waltz.
To keep the music playing.

ABOUT THE AUTHOR

Raz Shaw has been a theatre director for over twenty years and has directed plays all over the world from the South Bank to South Sudan. In 2016 he won Best Director at the UK Theatre Awards for his production of Margaret Edson's Pulitzer Prize-winning play *WIT*, about an American professor's battle with ovarian cancer. *Death and the Elephant* is his first book.

ACKNOWLEDGEMENTS

So many thanks. A mountain of gratitude.

To Brooke, whose spirit and courage (and brilliant book) inspired me to think about writing a book of my own in the first place.

To my first two readers, Naomi and Lucinda, for their wisdom, encouragement and, at times, fiercely honest notes.

To my 'sister' Louise, who was almost literally forced to read my first scribblings in a desperate bid for validation. Over the past three years she must have read the equivalent of a thousand pages. As ever she was wonderfully and (sometimes) painfully candid throughout. Her notes were always on the money. Thanks, Beans. A greater friend no man can have.

To all those others who were press-ganged into reading bits along the way and who gave me the confidence to keep going. You know who you are (aka I am scared to list people in case I miss somebody out!).

To Debbie, who was not only there by my side – cracking bad gags – from the cancer get-go and was (and still is) my rock, but who also gave me the two pieces of writing advice from which everything else followed:

a) Write for at least 30 minutes every day.
b) Don't get it right, get it written.

To my last reader, Julie Hes, for her endless support, the specificity of her notes and for her never-ending generosity. She's still annoying, mind you.

To my developmental editor, Tamsin Shelton, whose detailed brilliance helped give order and structure to a ragbag bunch of words.

To Mathew Clayton, who saw the potential in a random scattergun first draft and urged me to make significant changes whilst at no time making me feel he had lost faith in its potential. Without his backing, his support and insightful notes, this book would never have seen the light of day.

To John Mitchinson, whose force of personality alone gave me the impetus and courage to carry on just at the point when I had begun to doubt all that I was sure of (blatant Springsteen plagiarism right there!).

To Georgia Odd and Jimmy Leach, geniuses of crowdfunding, who dragged me kicking and screaming back onto social media and forced me to discover my inner American.

To DeAndra Lupu for her support, her wisdom, her empathy, her positivity, her sense of humour and her laser-like attention to every single detail. I spotted only one flaw. A blind eye to wonky tally marks. Nobody's perfect, I guess!

To Philip Connor and the rest of the Unbound family, most of whom I haven't even met, who have been beavering away tirelessly to make my book become just that. A book.

To Mark Bowsher for his gentle trailer-making magic.

To those who were by my side during the cancer days and are still by my side now. Tort and Tig and Al and Jo and Paul and Gesine and Mouse and Girsha and countless others. Your unwavering friendship and support back then gave me the strength to move forward when moving seemed the least likely option.

And, of course, to my family, most especially my mother, whose unconditional love and care has always been appreciated if not always expressed (by me). A stronger woman I have never known. She is even forgiven for introducing me to gambling.

And last but definitely not least, to all those whose generosity and support in pledging for this book repeatedly inspired me to keep on writing and re-writing and re-writing. I hope the end result has done you proud.

Thank you. Thank you. Thank you. Thank you. Thank you. Thank you.

SUPPORTERS

Unbound is a new kind of publishing house. Our books are funded directly by readers. This was a very popular idea during the late eighteenth and early nineteenth centuries. Now we have revived it for the internet age. It allows authors to write the books they really want to write and readers to support the books they would most like to see published.

The names listed below are of readers who have pledged their support and made this book happen. If you'd like to join them, visit www.unbound.com.

Roberta Aarons
Erica Stevens Abbitt
Anna Aleff
Michael Alexander
Esh Alladi
Diana Alter
Melanie Angell
Rosemary Ashe
Helen Ashton
Holly Augustine
Danni Bastian
Leon Baugh
Jason Baughan
Paul Beckett
Neil Beckett and
    Luciana Girotto
Natalie Beran

Vicky Berry
Charlotte Bevan
Larissa Bills
Giles Block
Sebastian Born
Kellie Bright
Deborah Bruce
Lotte Buchan
Bill & Siân Buckhurst
Niki Campbell
Sean Campion
Jo Carey
Lucy Carlson
Devalan Céline
Lorraine Cheesmur
Ceri-Lyn Cissone
Hannah Clark

Ollo Clark
Barbara Cohen
Neil Constable
Claire Cooper
Nikki Csànyi-Wills
Steph Curtis
James Dacre
Beth Daley
Brendan Davies
Naomi Dawson
Sarah Daykin
Emma Dhesi
Fia Dijksman
Sheila Dillon
Ryan Donaldson
Dominic Dromgoole
Diana Duke
Matthew Dunster
Isabelle Duperray
Sally Dynevor
Maggie Edson
Kate Ellis
Elaine Erny
Amber Evans
The Family Stone
Hayley Feigenbaum
Lea Ann Flanagan
Sue Flores
Louise Ford
Michael Ford
Hannah Fox
Phoebe Fox
Gail Francis

Tracey Fraser-Swatton
Terence Frisch
Jonathan Fuller
Marguerite Galizia
Georgia Gatti
Hilda Glumace
Claire Godden
Ellen Goodman
Jenny Grand
Steven Greenhalgh
Alasdair Greig
Alexandre Guansé
Damaris Gurney
Charlotte Hall
Clare Harding
Melissa Harrelson
Karen Harrison
Siubhan Harrison
Jack Hartnell
Mark Hayman
Renate Heitmann
Tatty Hennessy
Harry Hepple
Julie Hesmondhalgh
Jeremy Herrin
Sam Heughan
Rupert Hill
Helen Hillman
Lucy-Anne Holmes
Anthony Horowitz
Polly Hubbard
Madeleine Hutchins
Jasmine Hyde

Louie Ingham

Giulia Innocenti

Lucy Jackson

Matilda James

Nadia Jamil

Sabeen Jamil

Paul Jennings

Polly Jerrold

Krissy Jesudason

Janey Johnson

Farah Karim-Cooper

Dan Kieran

Brooke Kinsella

Anna Kirke

Jack Knowles

Eva Koch-Schulte

Sheila Kruze

Haruka Kuroda

Mia Lacey

Tiggy Lacey

George Lamb

David Lawrence

Helen Lawson

Pete Le May

Richard Lee

Tim Lee

Julie Legrand

Ambika Leigh

Luke Leighfield

Hanna Lingman

Lisa & Thomas

Jeremy Lloyd

Barney Luck

Jessica Lusk

Arshad Malik

Jayne Marshall

Abigail Matthews

Holly Matthews

Phil Mawer

Amy McCarthy

David McEvoy

Chris McGill

Jane McGinnes

Bruce McLeod

Caitlin McLeod

Tegan McLeod

Wendell McMurrain

Mark Melville

Adriana Mijaiche

Barbara Miller

Vicky Mills

Chris Milner

John Mitchinson

Laura Mitzman

Cam Moore

Jane Moriarty

Matt Morrison

Sarah Murray

Patrick Myles

Carlo Navato

Andrea Neumann-Claus

Jamie Newall

Emma Nicolson

Karen O'Toole

Sarah Oakes

Debbie Oates

Simone Rosa Ott
Tim Paige
Ria Paroubek-Groenewoud
Roz Perl
Nancy Perrelli
Alexis Peterman
Emma Pierson
Kate Plantin
Jenny Platt
Julia Platt
Justin Pollard
Samantha Power
Mark Quartley
Nicky Quint
Paula Rabbitt
Diane Rankin
Gwen Raphael
Maggie Rawlinson
Julia Redder
Ben Reid
Brenda and David Reid
Girsha Reid
Victoria Reid
Cathy Ritter
Ukweli Roach
Elizabeth Roberts
Sian Robins-Grace
Beatriz Romilly
Claudia Roncallo
Amy Rosenthal
Jasmine Rowe
Katherine Runnalls
Bernadette Russell

Charlie Russell
Luca Rutherford
Francesca Savige
Annette Scott
Jean Sergent
Ben Shaw
Brad Shaw
Katie Shaw
Mark & Michelle Shaw
Val Shaw
Henry Shields
Jayesh Sinha
Helen Siveter
Gesine Schmücker-Schüßler
Rich and Nia Smith
Jacqui Somerville
Ann Songhurst
Louise Spencer
M'artìna Spera
Mehul Srivastava
Kate Stafford
Leah Stephens
Naomi Stoll
Montgomery Sutton
Jessica Swale
Ben Tagoe
Tony Tassell
Giles Taylor
Melina Theocharidou
Adele Thomas
Rosie Townshend
Dan Usztan
Nathalie Vanderiet

Renee Veneziale
Johanna von Fischer
Laura Wade
Naomi Wallace
Chloe Walshe
Sacha Wares
Hannah Watkins
Pam Wayne
Georgie Weedon
Sarah Weltman
Lucinda Westcar

Amanda Whittington
Peter Wilkinson
Jade Williams
Lindsay Williams
Sian Williams
Jennie Cashman Wilson
Chris White
Amy Wolff
Sarah Woodward
Michelle Wormleighton
Tracy Zanelli